Please look for the following books by this author

A Different Approach to Hairbraiding: French Braiding and More

Braid Your Own Hair

Headband

Circle

Single

Double

Junction

Classic

Teardrop

Fringe

Crown

Halo

Heart

Acknowledgments

Without my models I would not have this book. Photos are important and essential.

Many people were a part of this book. I extend my thanks to each person for their invaluable help.

This book is dedicated to those who post online tutorials. Without that help none of my books would exist.

I invite you to join me in my approach to hairbraiding. It involves creating a hairstyle using three different components: Ways, Forms and Accents. This book is all about one of the Forms that I use and teach: Tails.

To learn all three components at the same time purchase
A Different Approach to Hairbraiding; French Braiding and More.

Hairstylist: Raychel Emmons
Design: Raychel Emmons
Graphics: Raychel Emmons
Photography: Raychel Emmons
Photoshop: Raychel Emmons

Braider Creator, Book and App

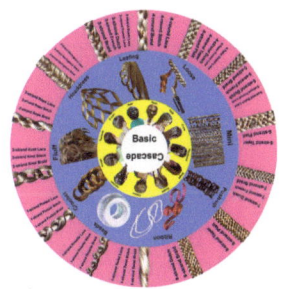

1. Line up the arrow on the Braider Creator.

   (The Braider Creator is available for download on my website www.findingbraids.com. It is a device that points out hairstyles but it does not show the finished results. You must envision the final results. Each of you will come up with different versions of the same style.

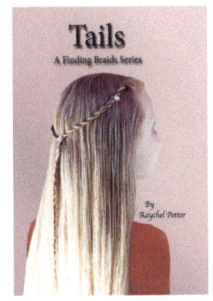

2. Use this book and your imagination to learn how to create hundreds of examples of that style.

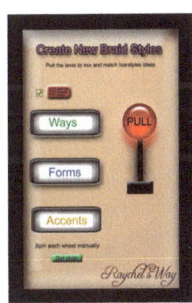

3. Take a well lit photo of each example you create and load it into the Finding Braids App. By doing this you will become a contributor to a world wide database of braids.

   Repeat! This is the essence of Raychel's Way.

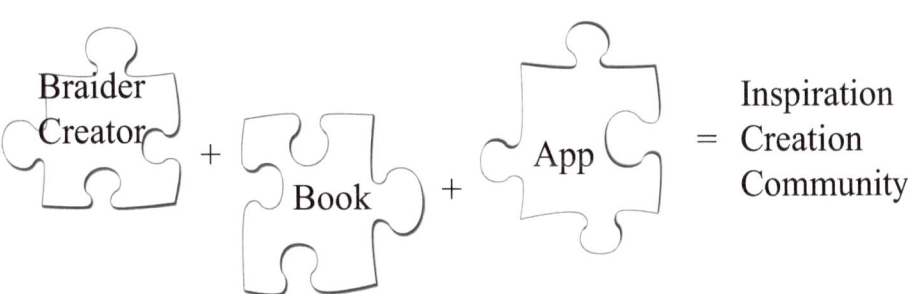

Braider Creator + Book + App = Inspiration Creation Community

Kinds of Braids

Here are the kinds of braids that I know.
You may apply them to the tail form to create different hairstyles.

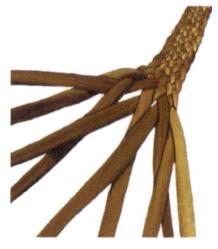

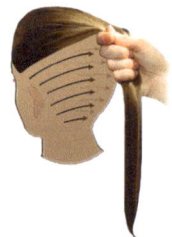

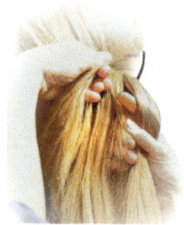

Braid = no gathers

(A braid can hang
loose or pin up into a
bun. Be creative!)

Stitch = gather into
both sides of the braid.

(Leave the tail long or pin it
into a bun.)

Lace = gather into one
side of the braid.

(Many types of lace braids will
unravel if the tail is not pinned
into a bun.)

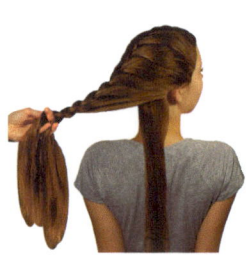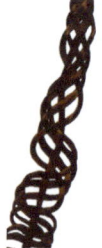

Feather Loose = holding the
braid away from the head while
you braid to create a loose braid
or opening and loosening a tight
braid to create filigree.

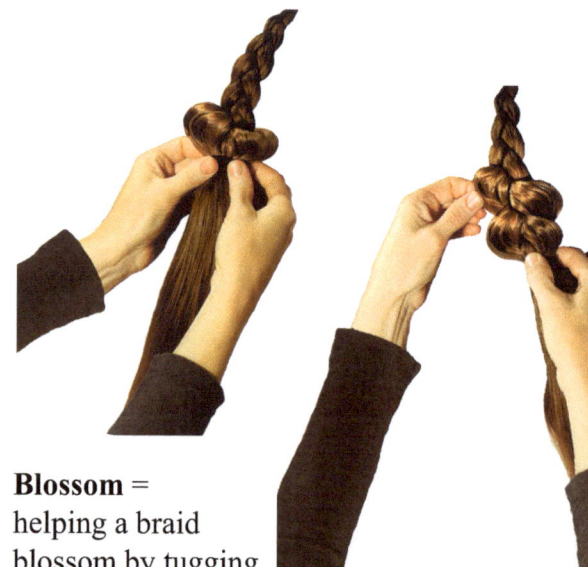

Blossom =
helping a braid
blossom by tugging
out the pedals of each braid bump until it looks like
a flower in full bloom.

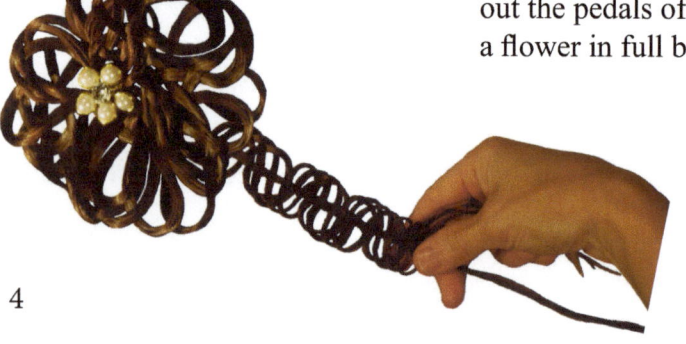

Push Up = pushing up all but one
strand of the braid to create a flower
or celtic design.

4

Stitching a Tail

Tails may be stitched with any number of strands. Each number adds it's own unique beauty to the tail. A tail may be stitched in the following three ways:

Symmetrically in the front to create a cage pattern around the tail.

In a spiral to create a spiraling staircase pattern.

On each side.

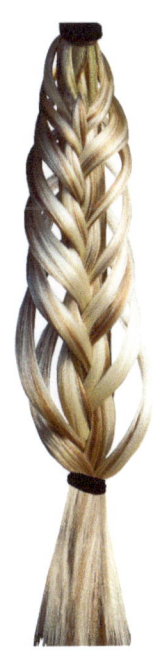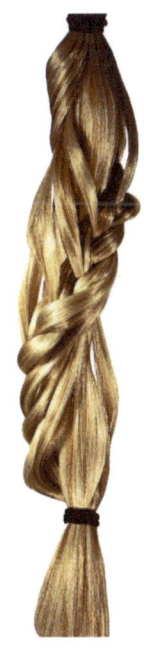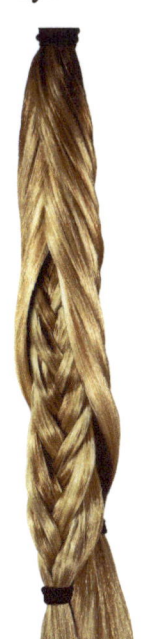

Lacing a Tail

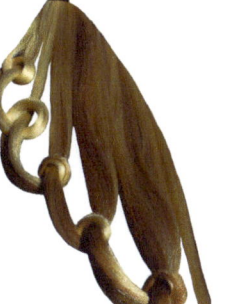

Tails may be laced with any number of strands. Each number adds it's own unique beauty to the tail. A tail may be laced in the following three ways:

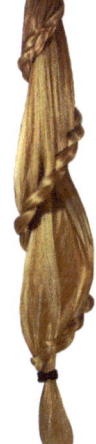

Symmetrically on each side.

On only one side.

In a spiral to create a spiraling staircase pattern.

Table of Contents

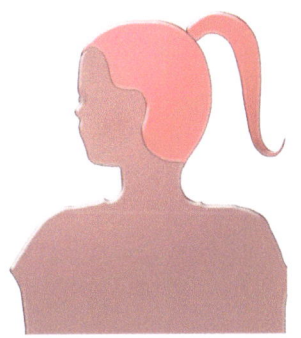

Basic   Pages 11-33

Make one tail or make 100 tails. It doesn't matter where you place the braids as long as all of the hair is used.

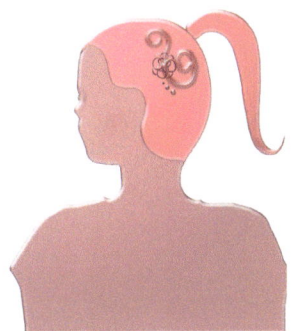

Accent   Pages 35-53

Make one tail or make 100 tails. It doesn't matter where you place the braids as long as all of the hair is used. Accents differ from basics by leaving out slivers of hair to create accents. Accents add a decorative flare to any hairstyle including just a plain old unbraided ponytail.

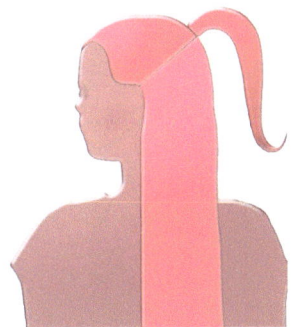

Cascade   Pages 55-67

Make one tail or make 100 tails. It doesn't matter where you place the braids as long as half of the hair is left out.

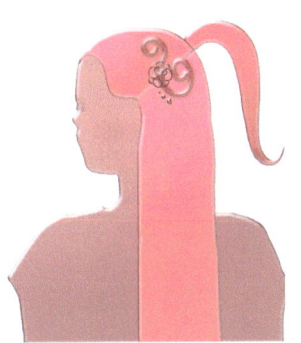

Accent Cascade   Pages 69-79

Make one tail or make 100 tails. It doesn't matter where you place the braids as long as half of the hair is left out. One or several slivers of hair are used to create accents. Accents add a decorative flare to any hairstyle including just a plain old unbraided ponytail.

Basic Tails

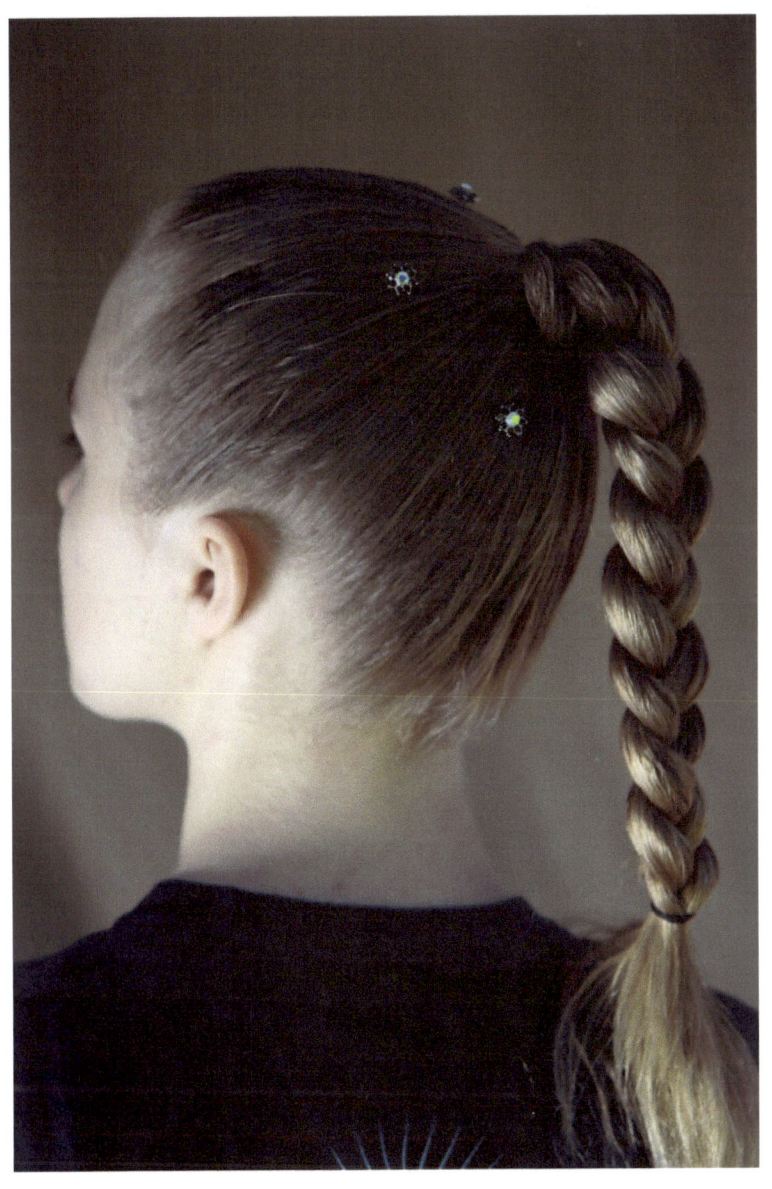

Basic Tail Placement

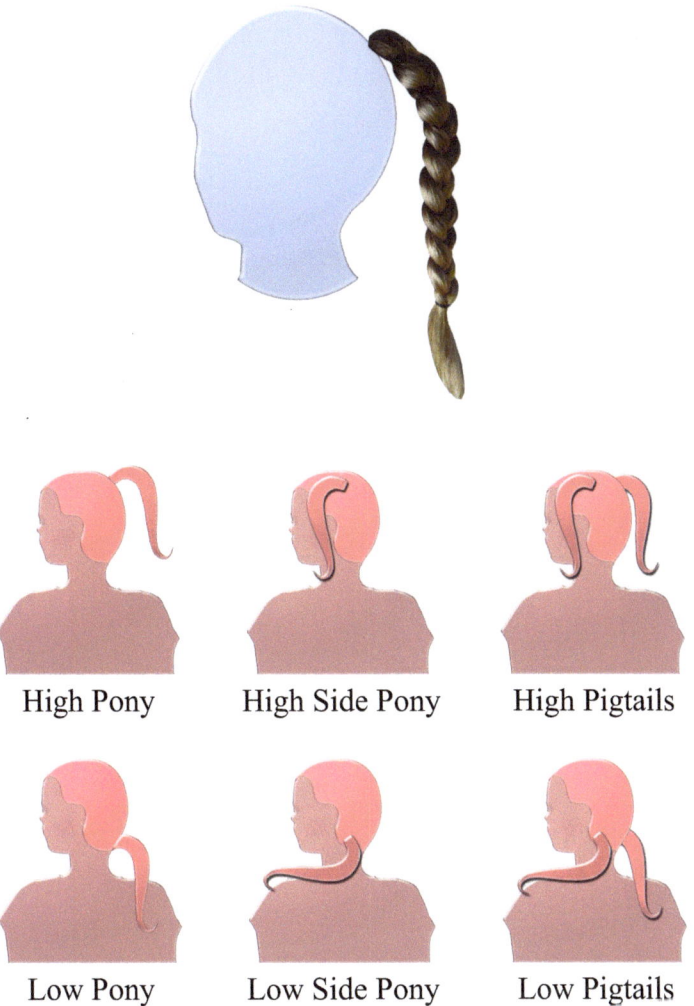

High Pony   High Side Pony   High Pigtails

Low Pony   Low Side Pony   Low Pigtails

The Icons above are suggestions of a few common placements for a basic tail. The basic tail is already incredibly versatile even before we start talking about braiding. How many more placements can you think of that I have not suggested? Can you imagine how thick this book would be if I showed each one? It would take me ten years to write and I already spent ten years writing the first book. So, I will make this a small book and I will let you use your imagination and creativity to come up with the other placements.

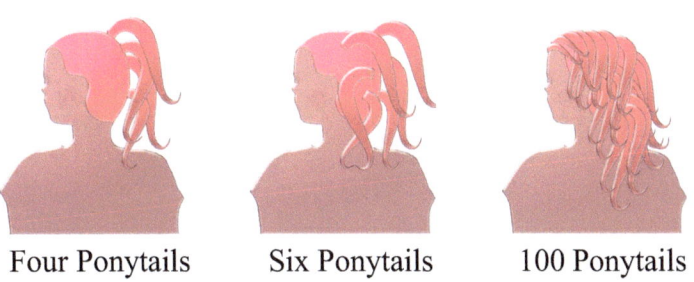

Four Ponytails   Six Ponytails   100 Ponytails

Basic

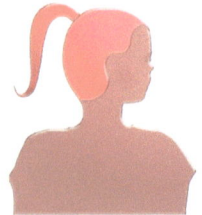

Make one tail or make 100 tails. It doesn't matter where you place the braids as long as all of the hair is used.

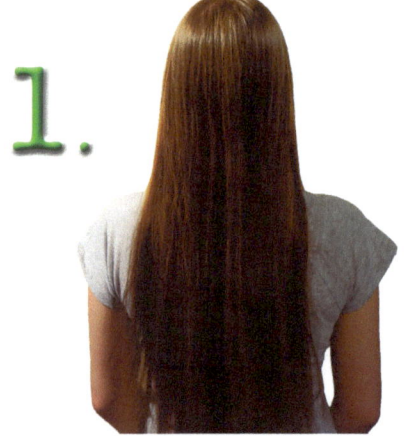

1.

Begin with clean, brushed hair.

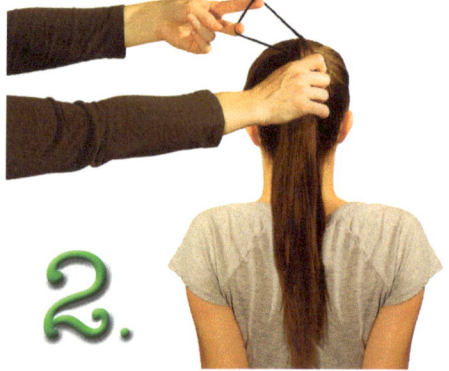

2.

The High Ponytail is the first example. Use a covered rubber band to place all the hair into a ponytail.

All the examples below are High Ponytails. Some are just the tail braided, some are the braid pinned up into a bun, and some are multiple braids pinned up.

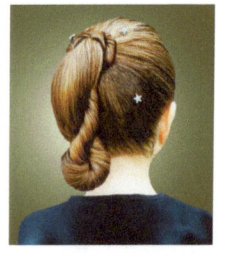
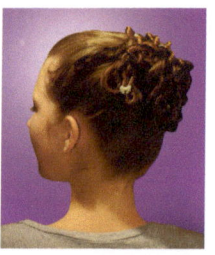
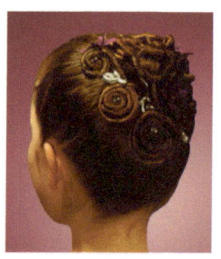
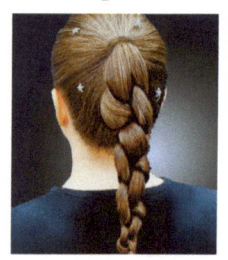
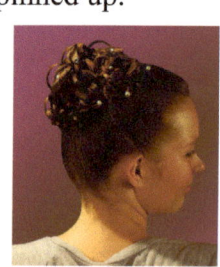

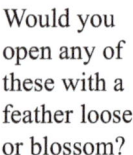
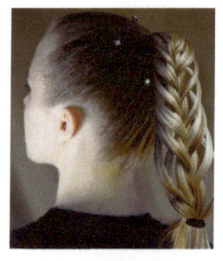
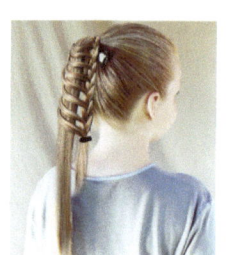
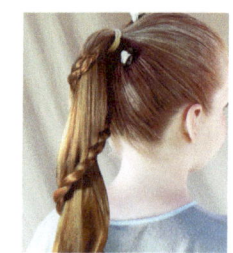
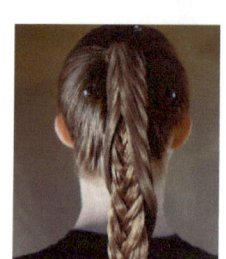

Would you open any of these with a feather loose or blossom?

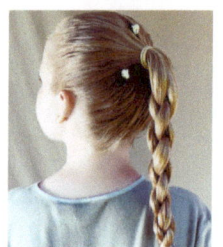
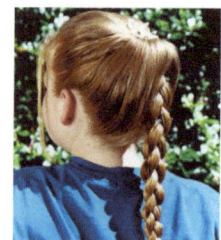
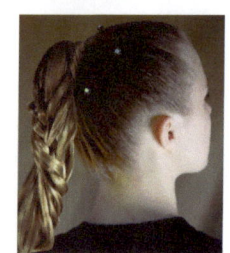
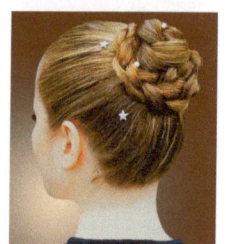

Basic

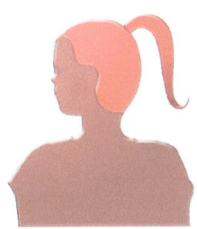

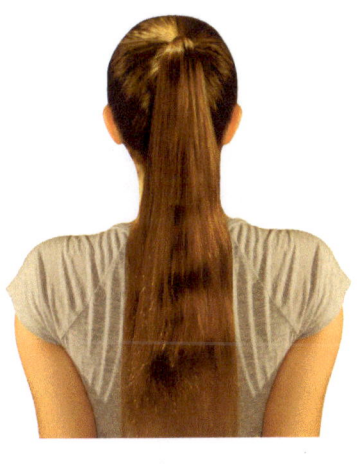

3. Once the ponytail is placed right where you want it, choose a number of strands to braid with.

After the number of strands has been chosen, decide how many braids will be made.

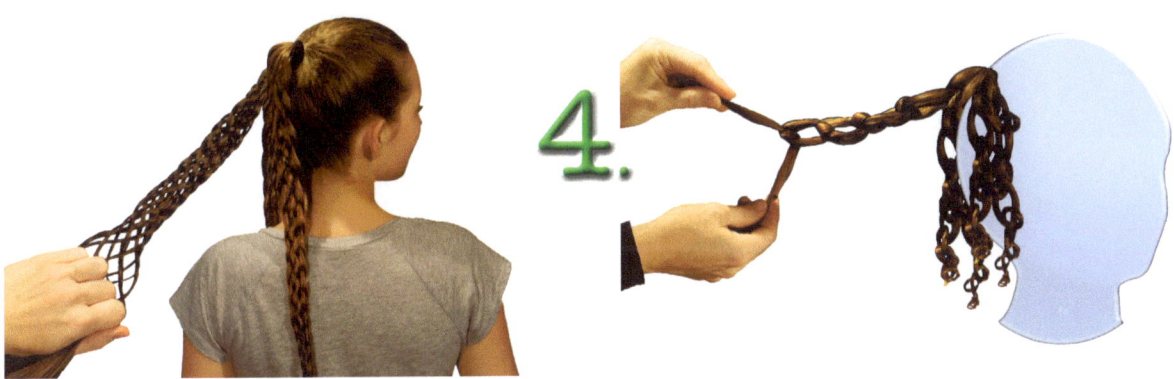

4.

Finally, determine if those braids will hang down or be pinned up.

5.

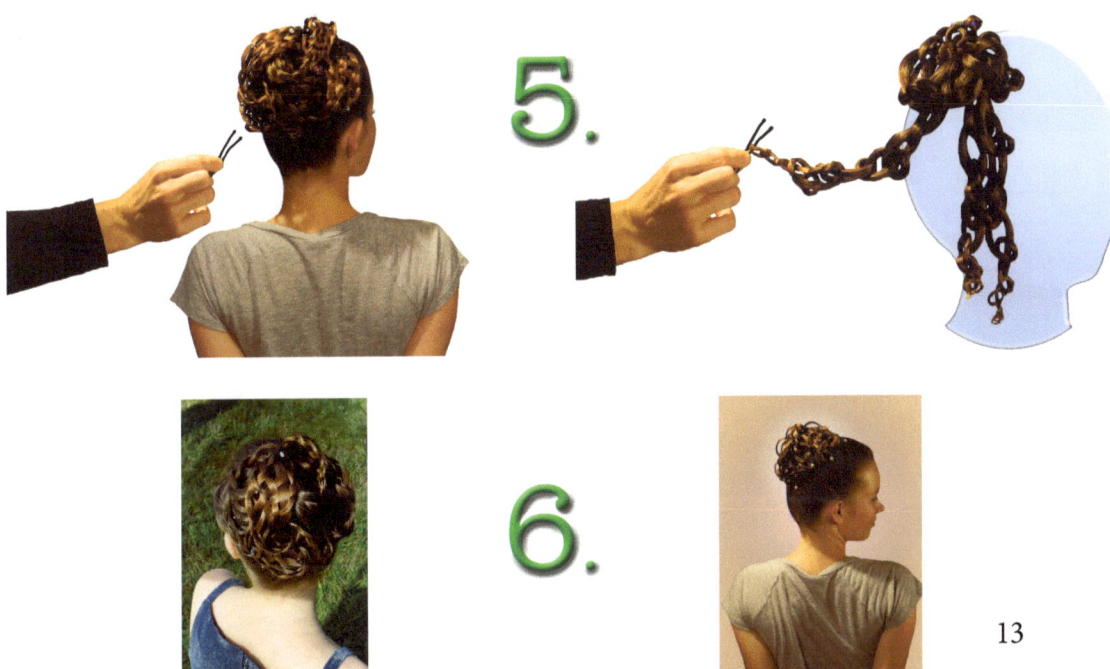

6.

13

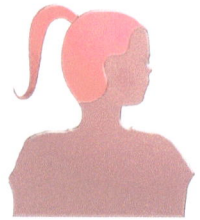

Basic

Make one tail or make 100 tails. It doesn't matter where you place the braids as long as all of the hair is used.

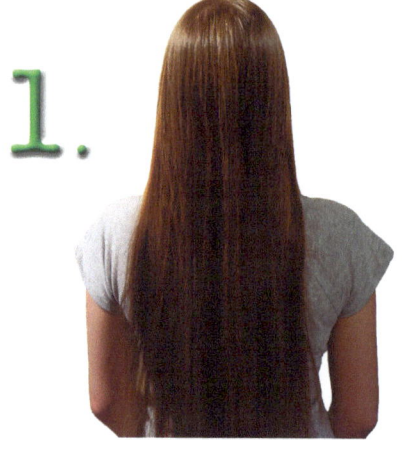

1.

Begin with clean, brushed hair.

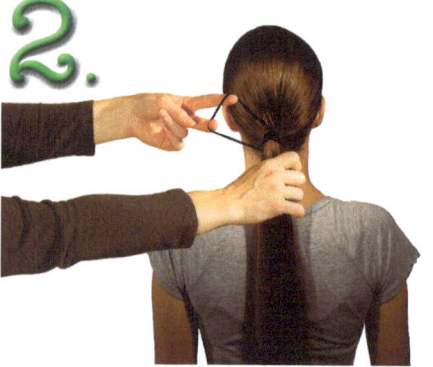

2.

Use a covered rubber band to place all the hair into a ponytail. I am placing a Low Ponytail

All the examples below are Low Ponytails. Some are just the tail braided, some are the braid pinned up into a bun.

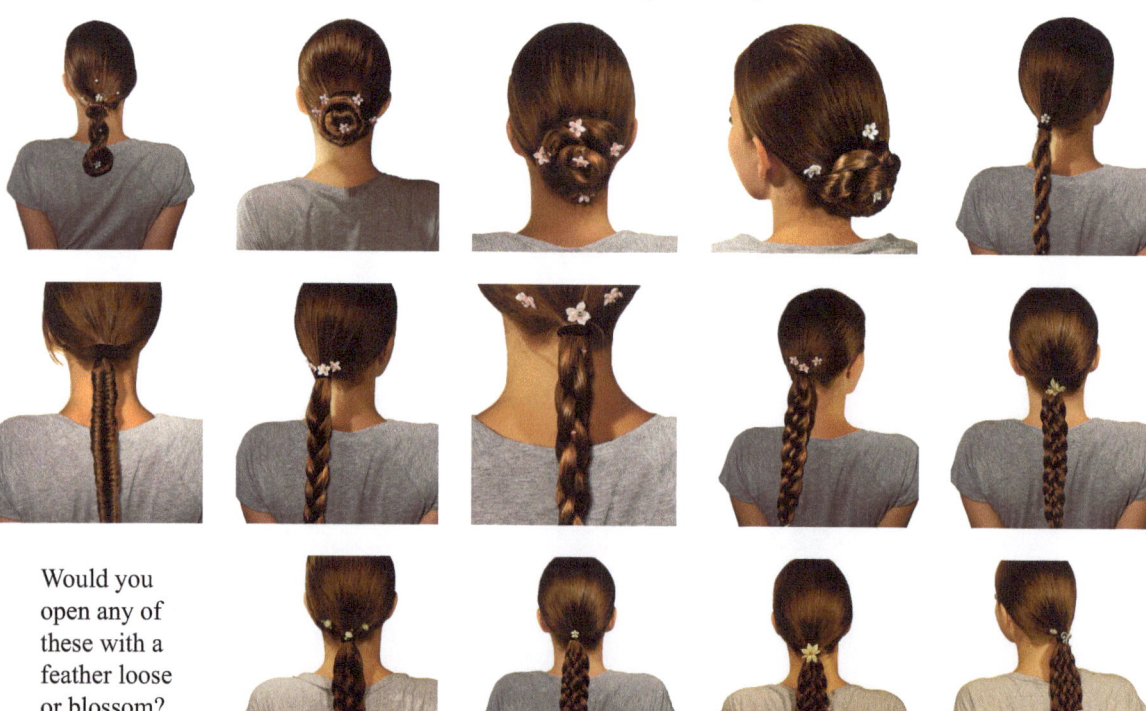

Would you open any of these with a feather loose or blossom?

Basic

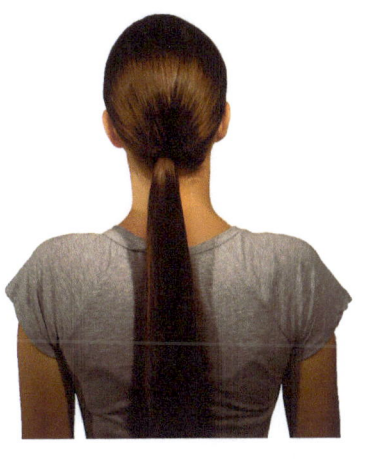

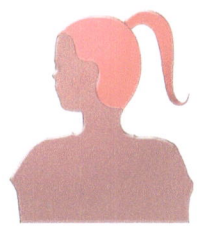

3. Once the ponytail is placed right where you want it, choose a number of strands to braid with.

After the number of strands has been chosen, decide how many braids will be made.

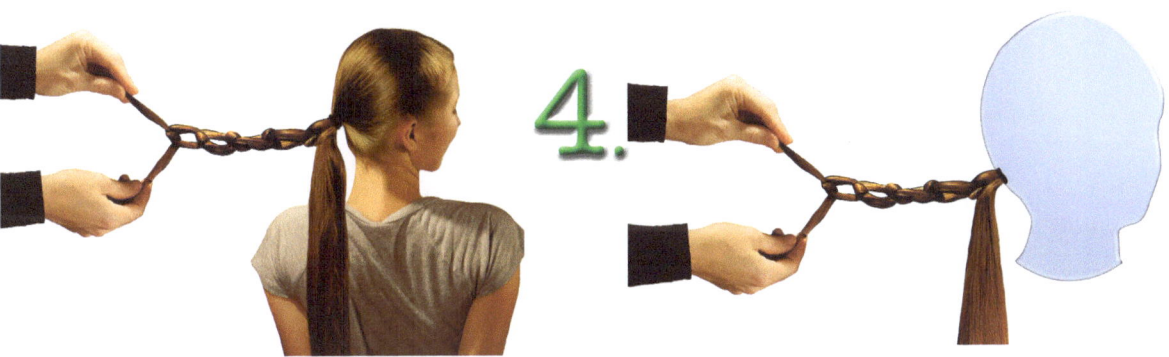

4.

Finally, determine if those braids will hang down or be pinned up.

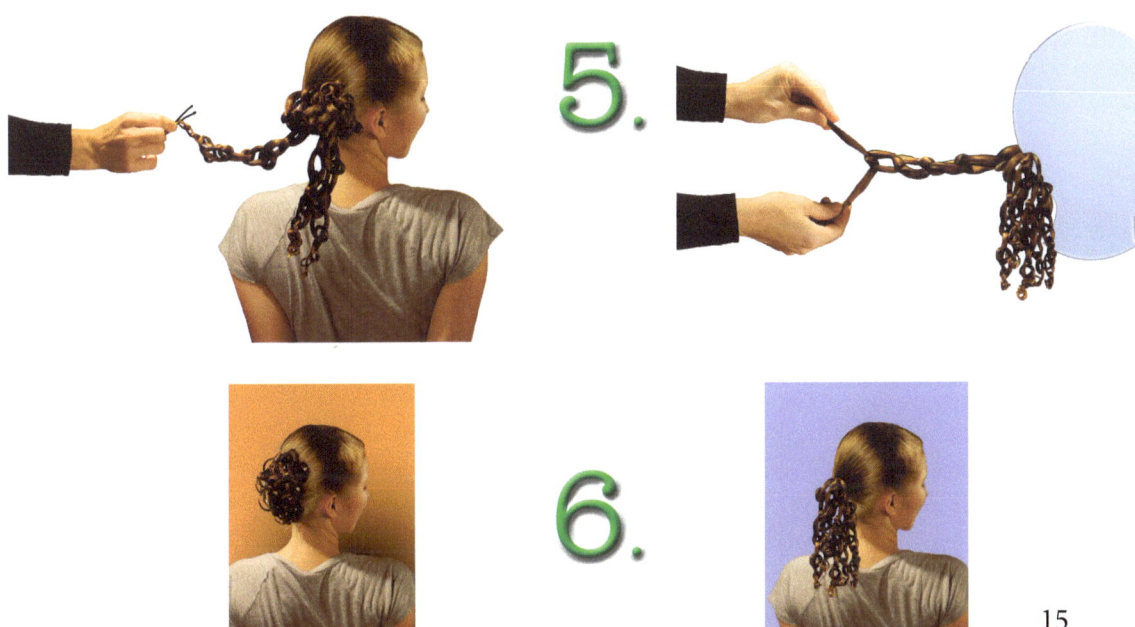

5.

6.

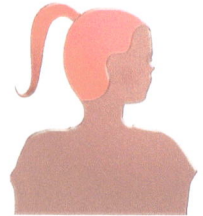

Basic

Make one tail or make 100 tails. It doesn't matter where you place the braids as long as all of the hair is used.

1.

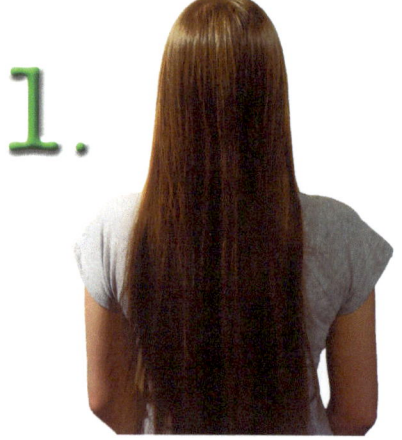

Begin with clean, brushed hair.

2.

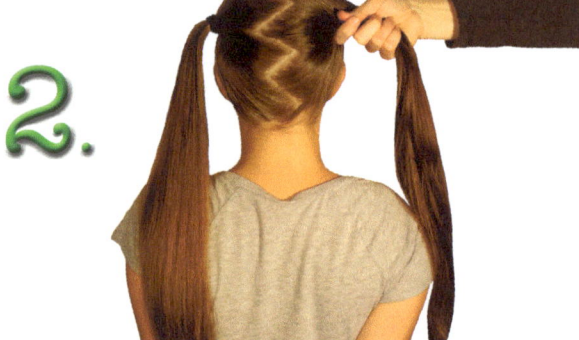

Use a covered rubber band to place all the hair into ponytails. I am placing High Pigtails

All the examples below are High Pigtails. Some are just the tails braided, some are the braids pinned up into buns, and some are multiple braids from each ponytail.

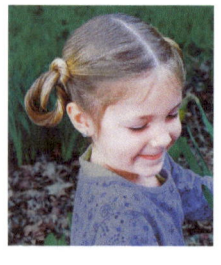
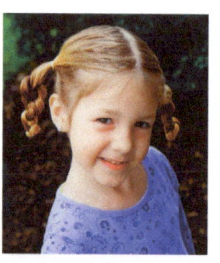
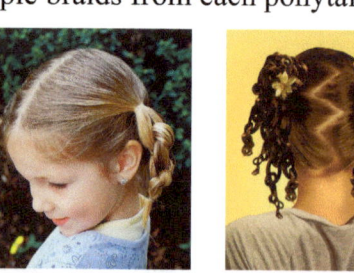

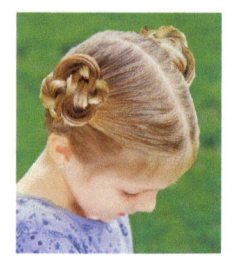
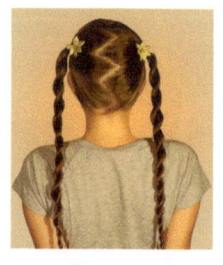
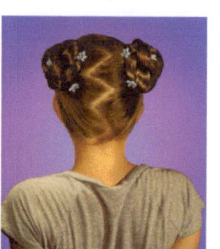
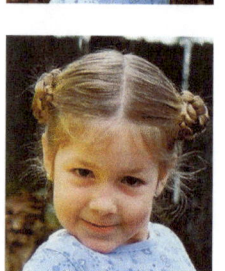
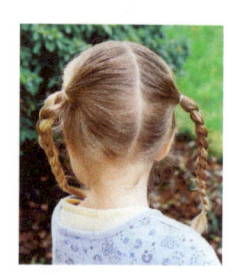

Would you open any of these with a feather loose or blossom?

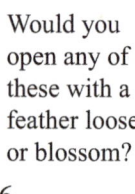
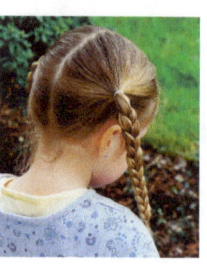
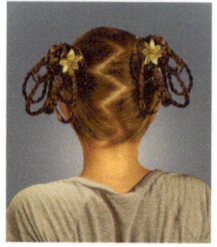
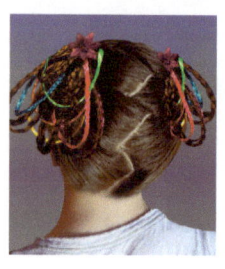
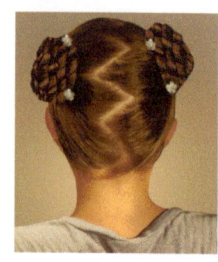

16

Basic

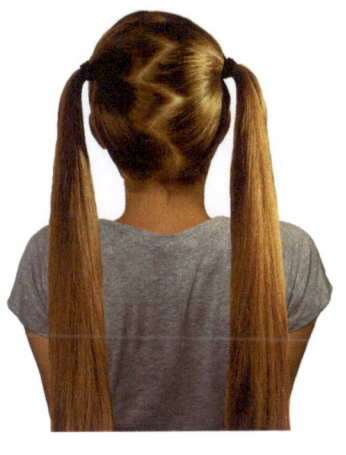

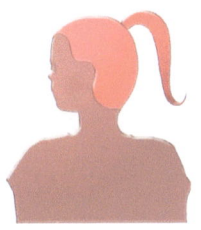

3.
Once the ponytails are placed right where you want them, choose a number of strands to braid with.

After the number of strands has been chosen, decide how many braids will be made.

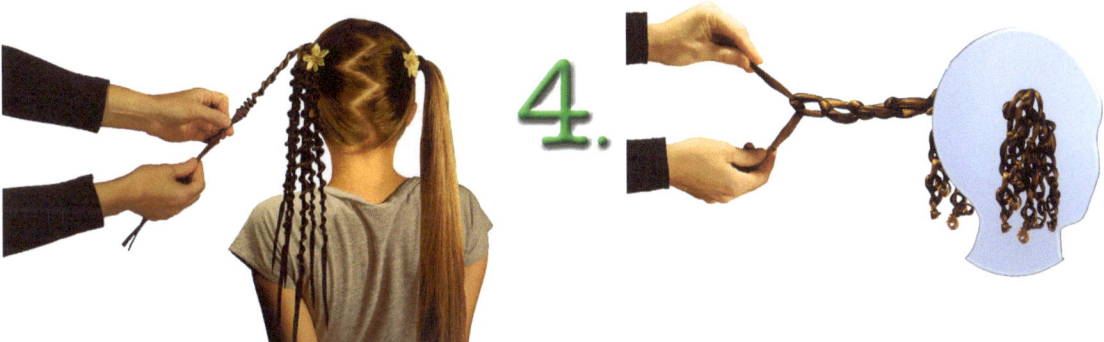

4.

Finally, determine if those braids will hang down or be pinned up.

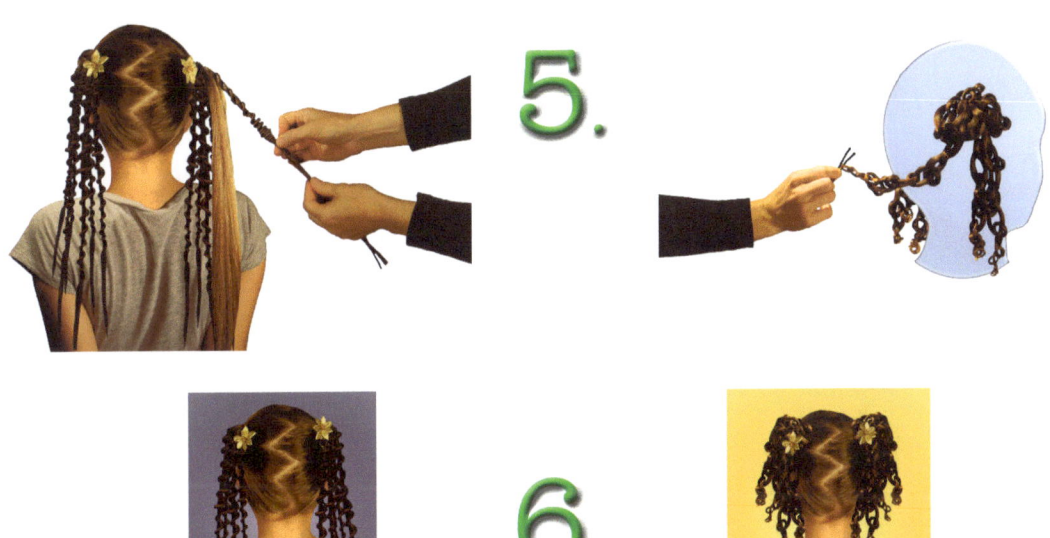

5.

6.

Basic

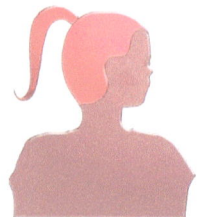

Make one tail or make 100 tails. It doesn't matter where you place the braids as long as all of the hair is used.

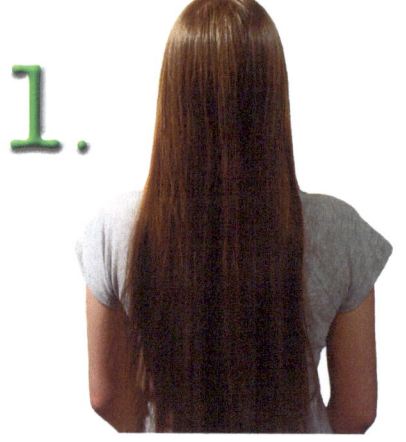

1.

Begin with clean, brushed hair.

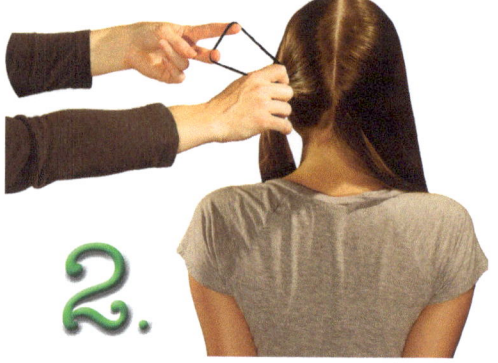

2.

Use a covered rubber band to place all the hair into ponytails. I am placing Low Pigtails

All the examples below are Low Pigtails. Some are just the tails braided, some are the braids pinned up into buns, and some are multiple braids from each ponytail.

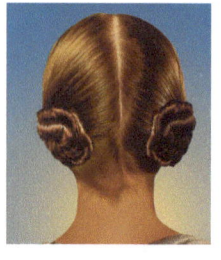
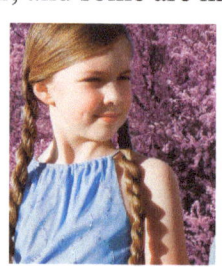
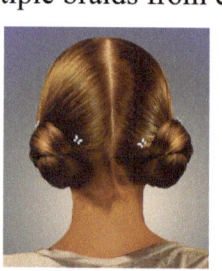
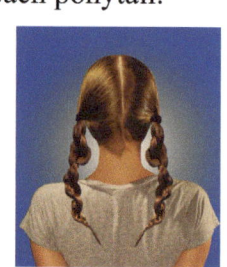

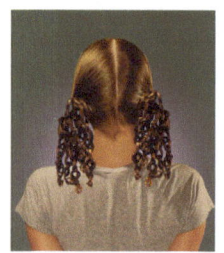
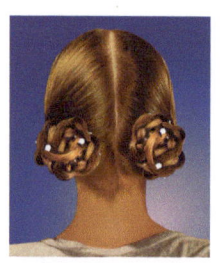
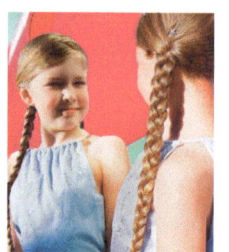
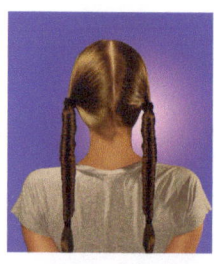
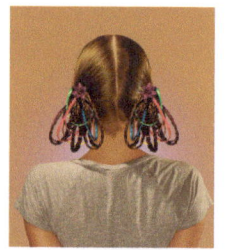

Would you open any of these with a feather loose or blossom?

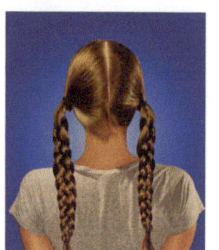
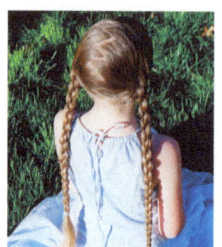
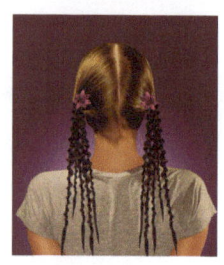
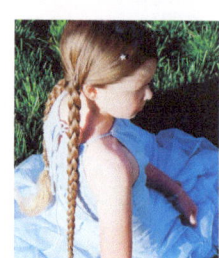

18

Basic

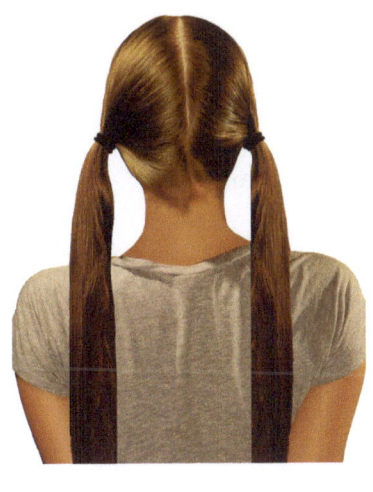

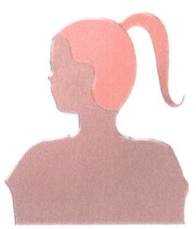

3. Once the ponytails are placed right where you want them, choose a number of strands to braid with.

After the number of strands has been chosen, decide how many braids will be made.

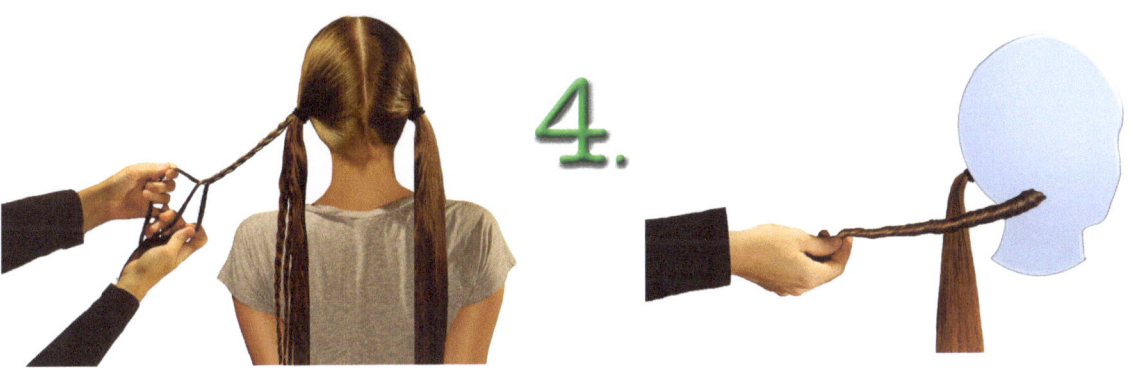

4.

Finally, determine if those braids will hang down or be pinned up.

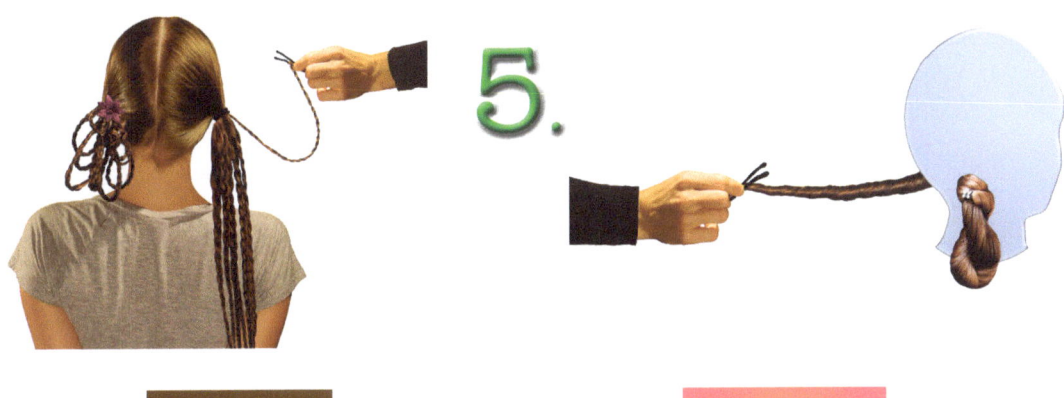

5.

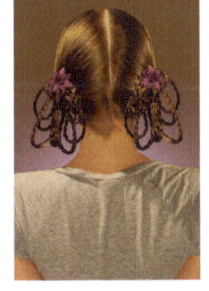

6.

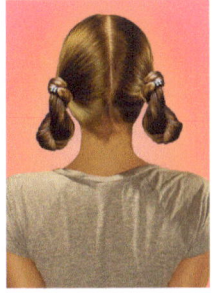

Basic

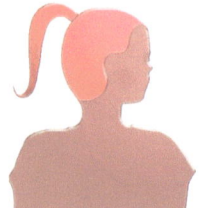

Make one tail or make 100 tails. It doesn't matter where you place the braids as long as all of the hair is used.

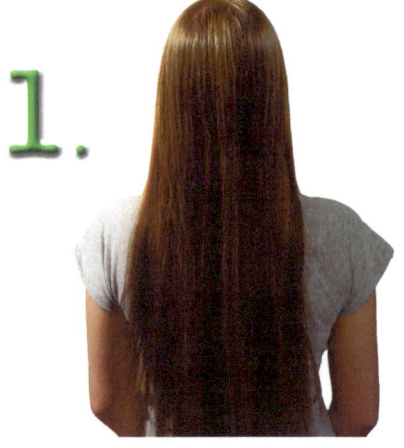

1.

Begin with clean, brushed hair.

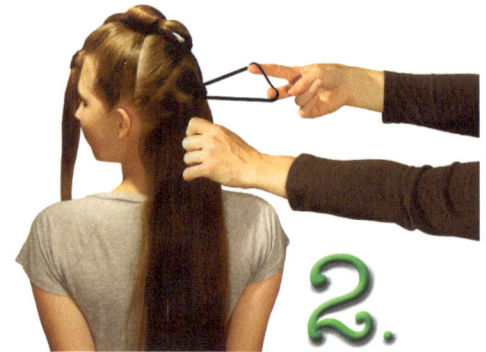

2.

Use a covered rubber band to place all the hair into ponytails. I am placing four ponytails where a mohawk typically resides.

All the examples below are four Ponytails. Some are just the tails braided, some are the braids pinned up into buns, and some are multiple braids from each ponytail.

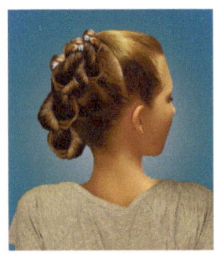 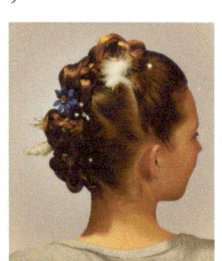 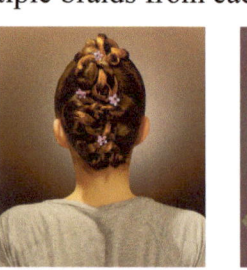 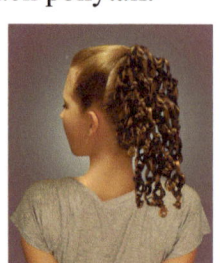

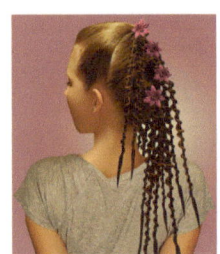 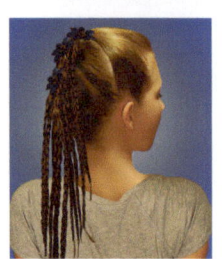 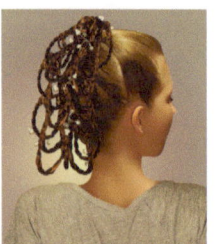 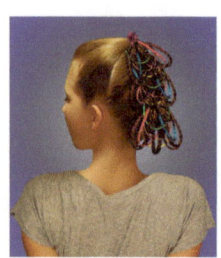 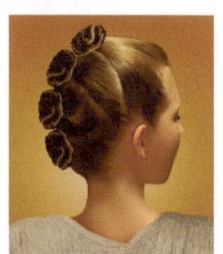

Would you open any of these with a feather loose or blossom?

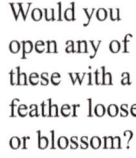 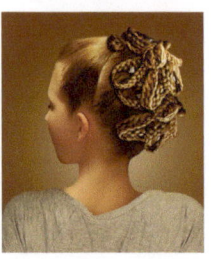 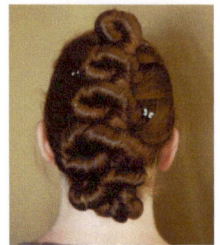 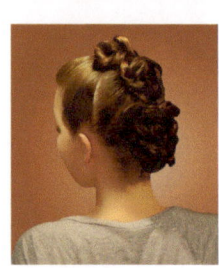 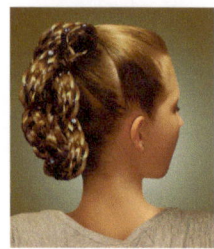

Basic

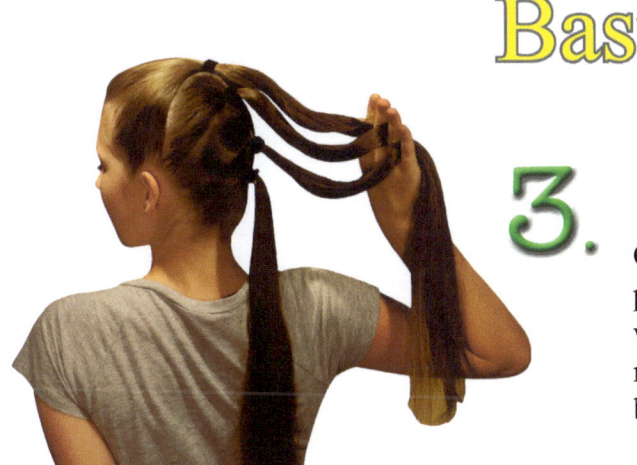

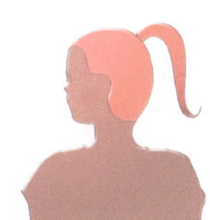

3.

Once the ponytails are placed right where you want them, choose a number of strands to braid with.

After the number of strands has been chosen, decide how many braids will be made.

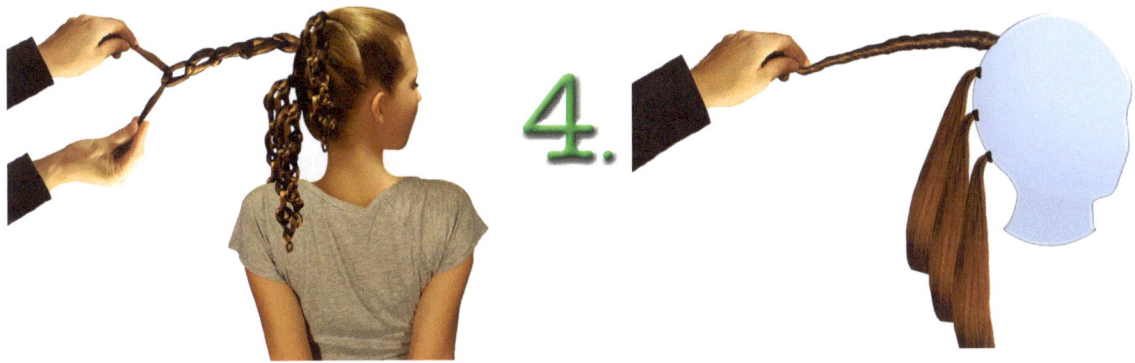

4.

Finally, determine if those braids will hang down or be pinned up.

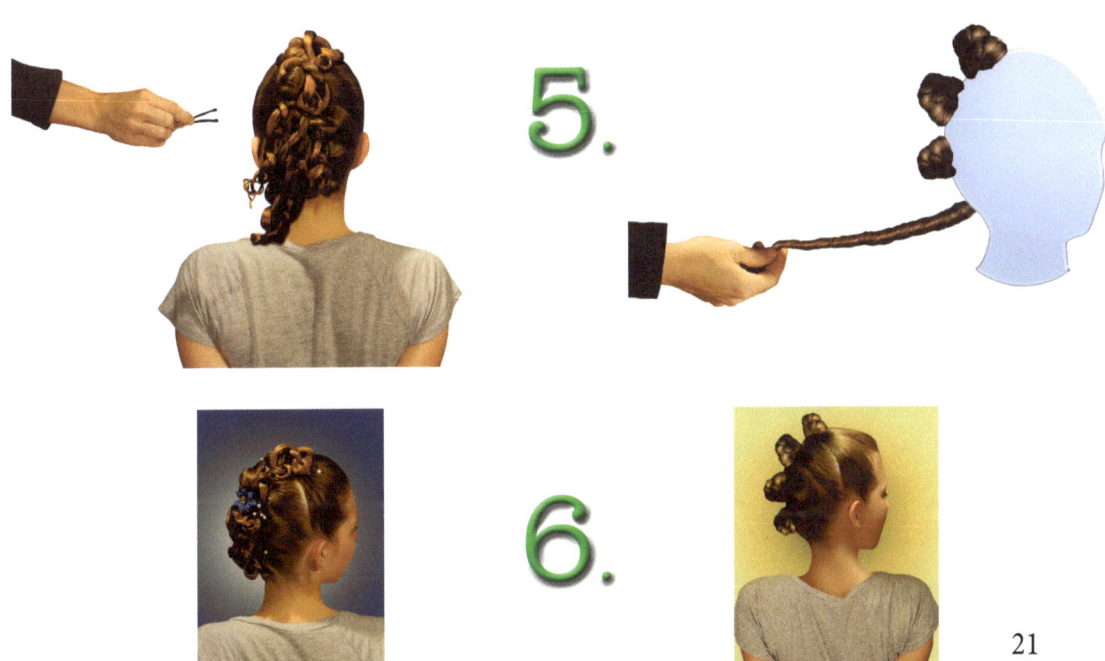

5.

6.

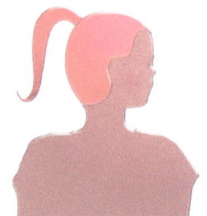

Basic

Make one tail or make 100 tails. It doesn't matter where you place the braids as long as all of the hair is used.

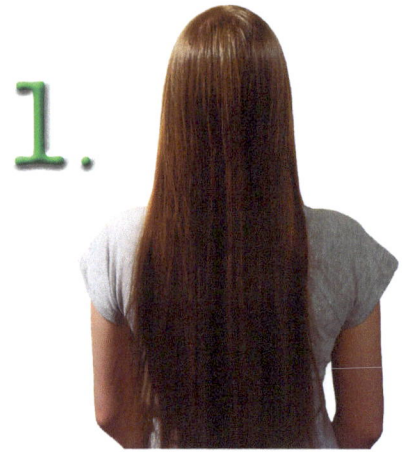

1.

Begin with clean, brushed hair.

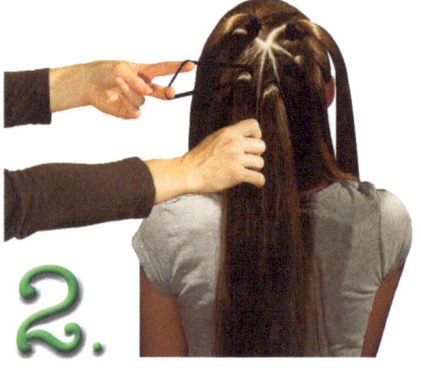

2.

Use a covered rubber band to place all the hair into ponytails. I am placing ponytails in multiple locations.

All the examples below use more than one ponytail. Some are just the tail braided, some are the braid pinned up into a bun, and some are multiple braids from each ponytail.

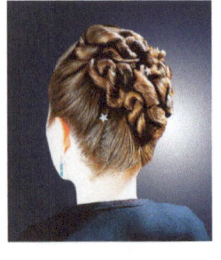
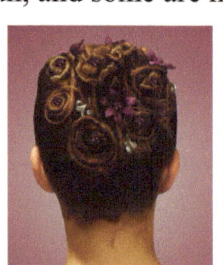
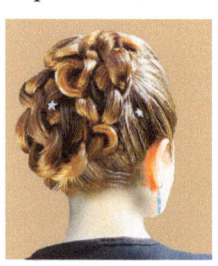
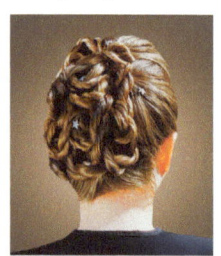

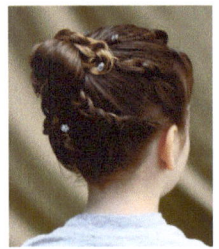
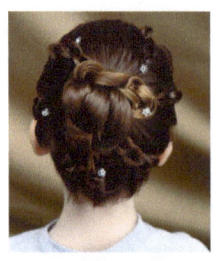
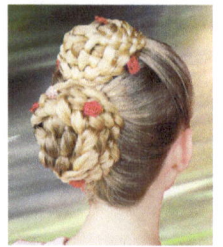
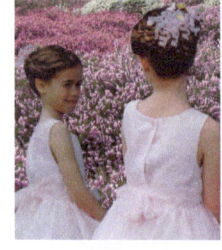
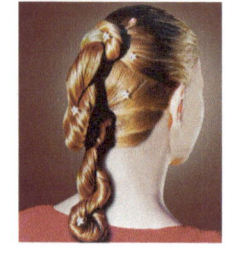

Would you open any of these with a feather loose or blossom?

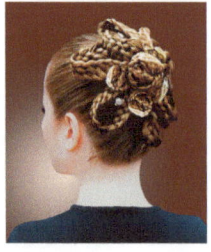
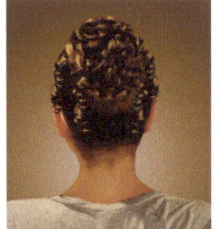
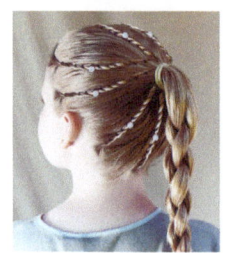

Basic

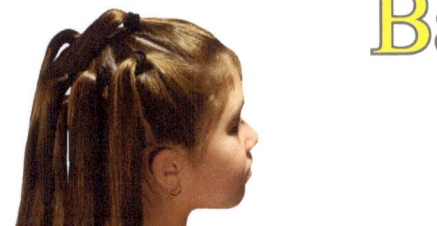

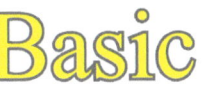

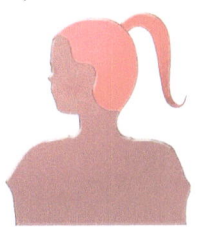

3. Once the ponytails are placed right where you want them, choose a number of strands to braid with.

After the number of strands has been chosen, decide how many braids will be made.

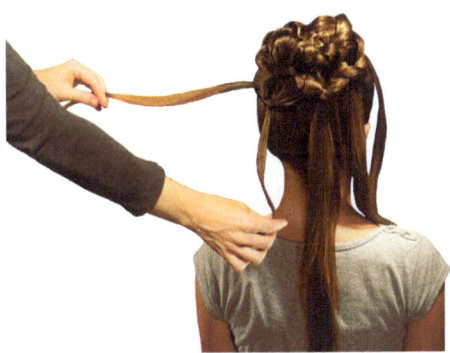

4.

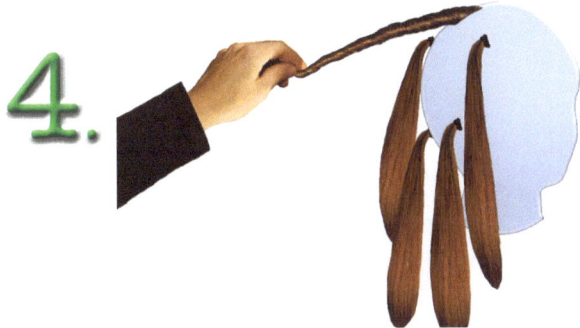

Finally, determine if those braids will hang down or be pinned up.

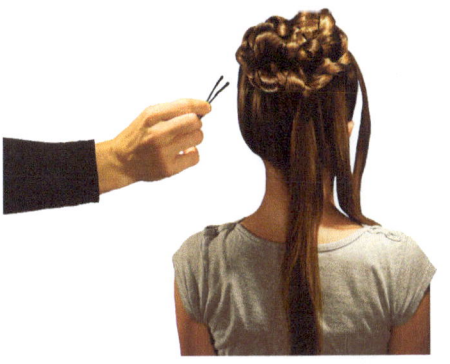

5.

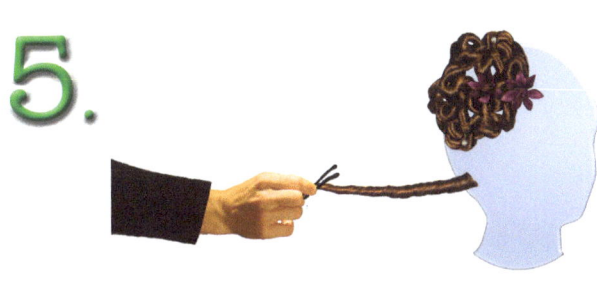

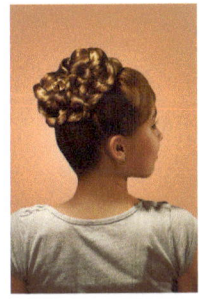

6.

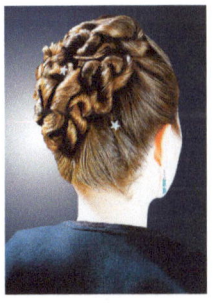

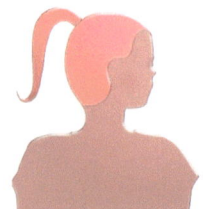

Basic

Make one tail or make 100 tails. It doesn't matter where you place the braids as long as all of the hair is used.

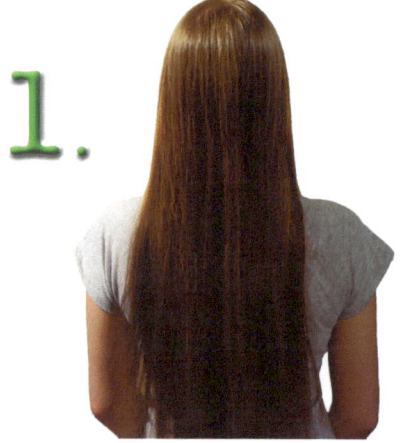

Begin with clean, brushed hair.

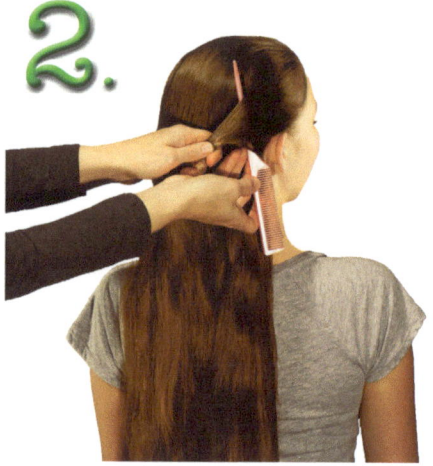

I am placing dozens of ponytails.

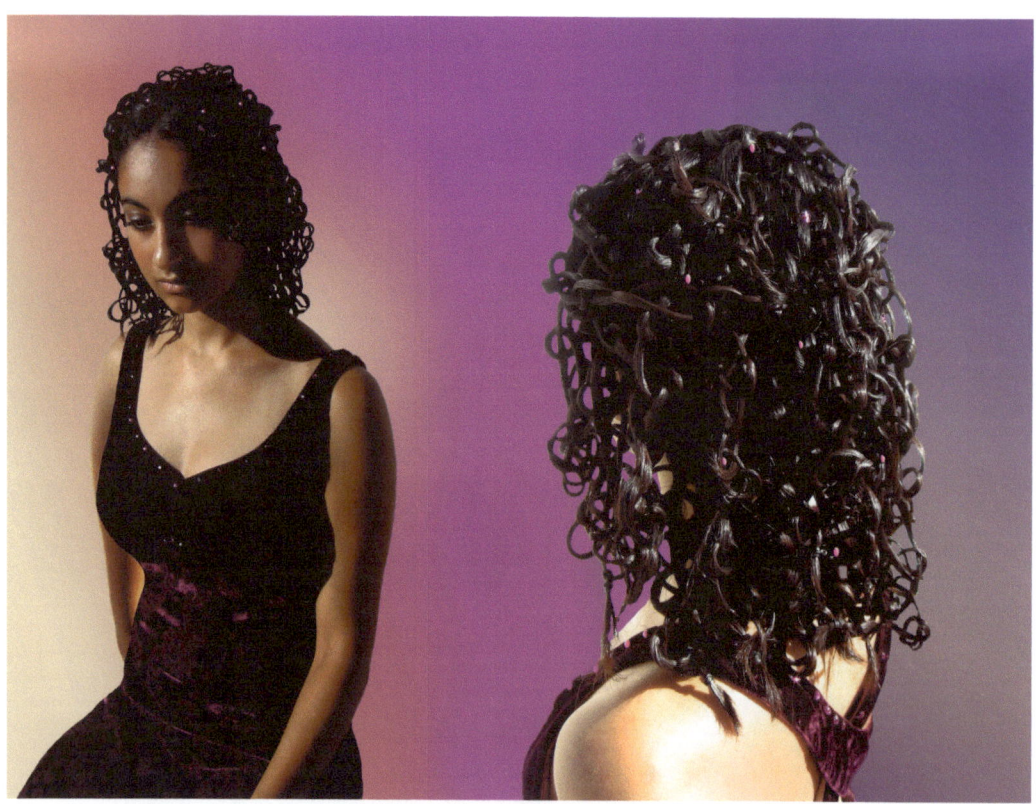

Basic

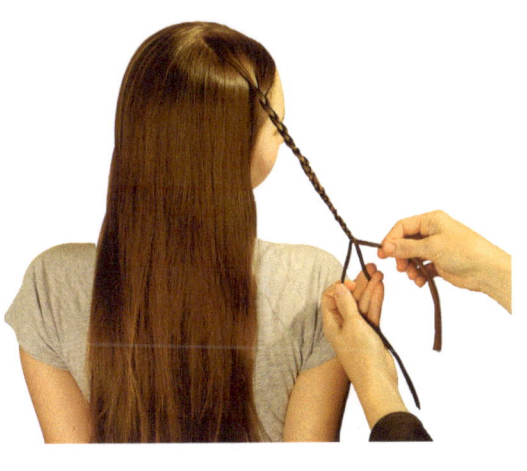
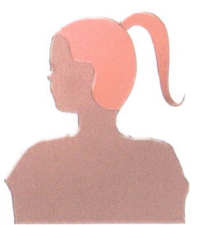

3.
Once the ponytails are placed right where you want them, choose a number of strands to braid with.

After the number of strands has been chosen, decide how many braids will be made.

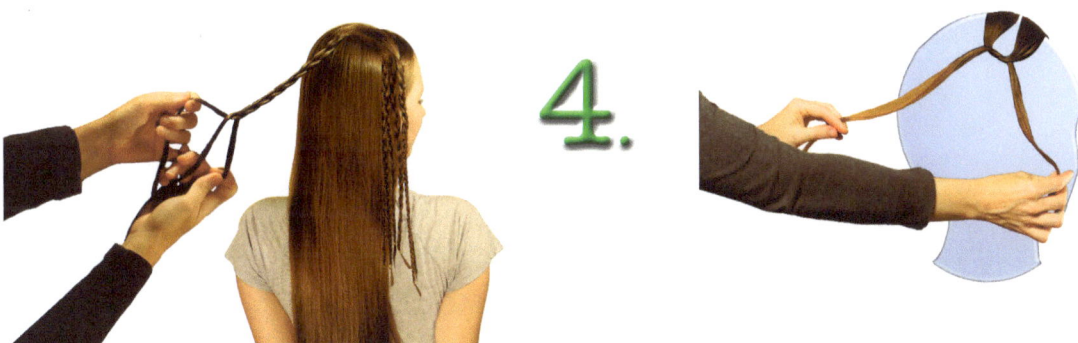

4.

Finally, determine if those braids will hang down or be pinned up.

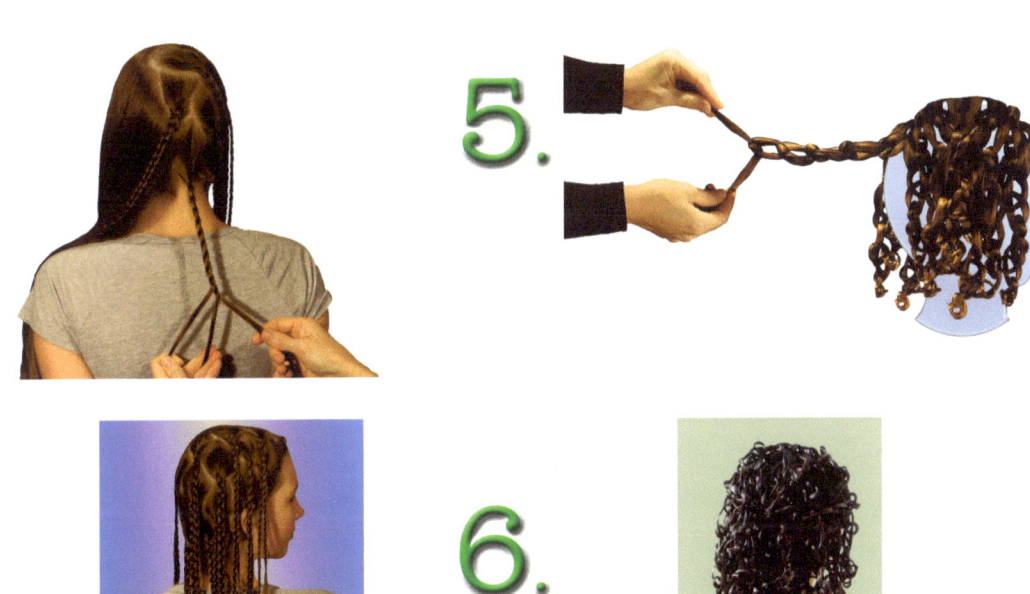

5.

6.

Basic

Make one tail or make 100 tails. It doesn't matter where you place the braids as long as all of the hair is used.

1.

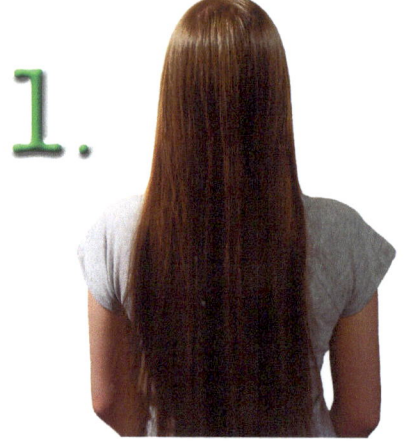

Begin with clean, brushed hair.

2.

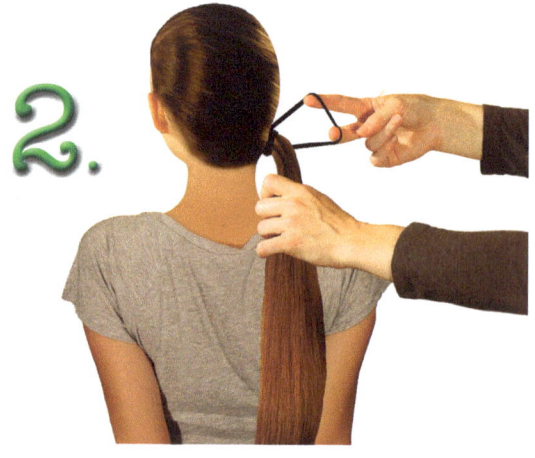

I am placing a side ponytail.

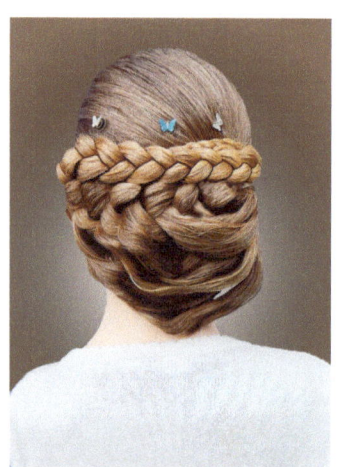

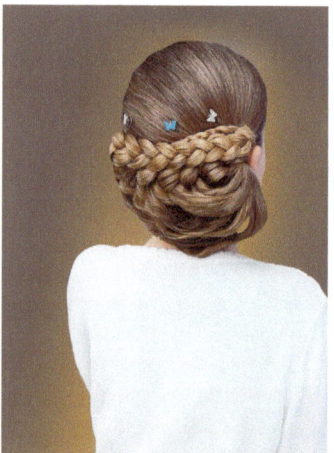

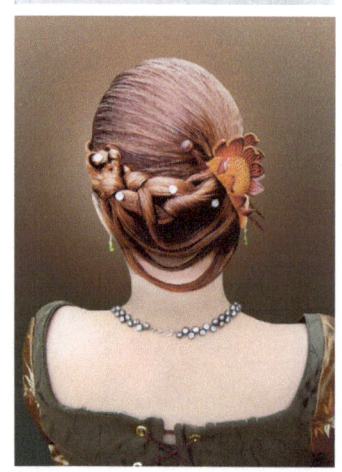

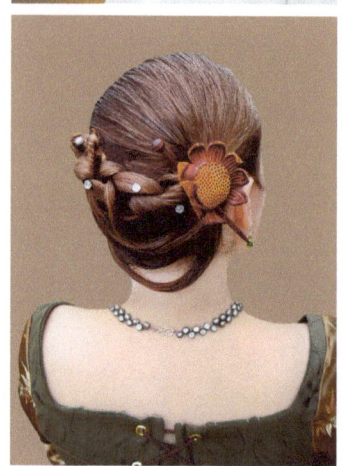

Basic

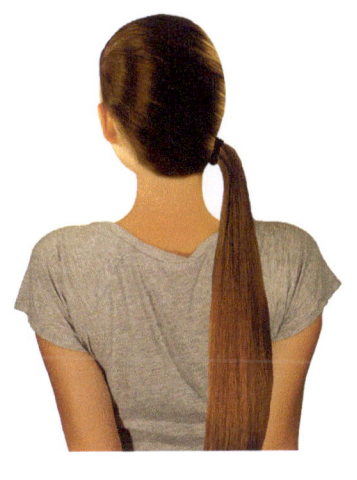

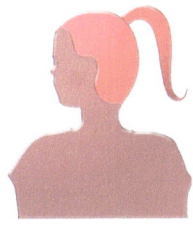

3. Once the ponytail is placed right where you want it, choose a number of strands to braid with.

After the number of strands has been chosen, decide how many braids will be made.

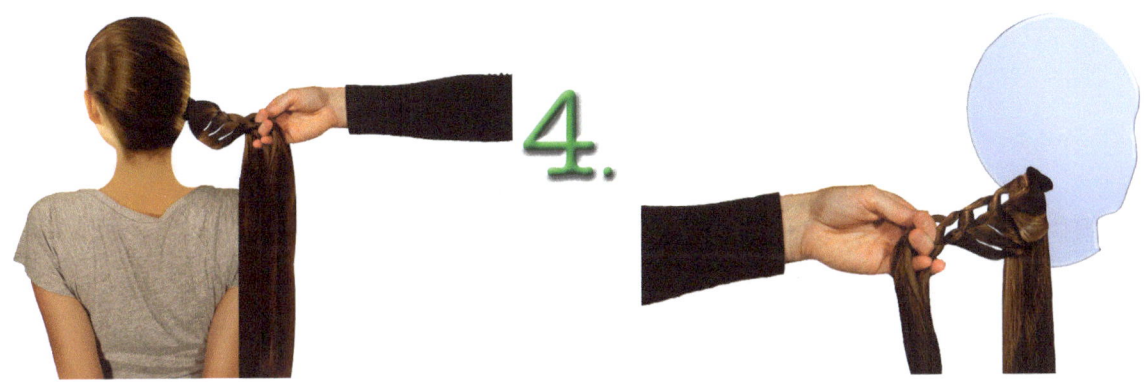

4.

Finally, determine if those braids will hang down or be pinned up.

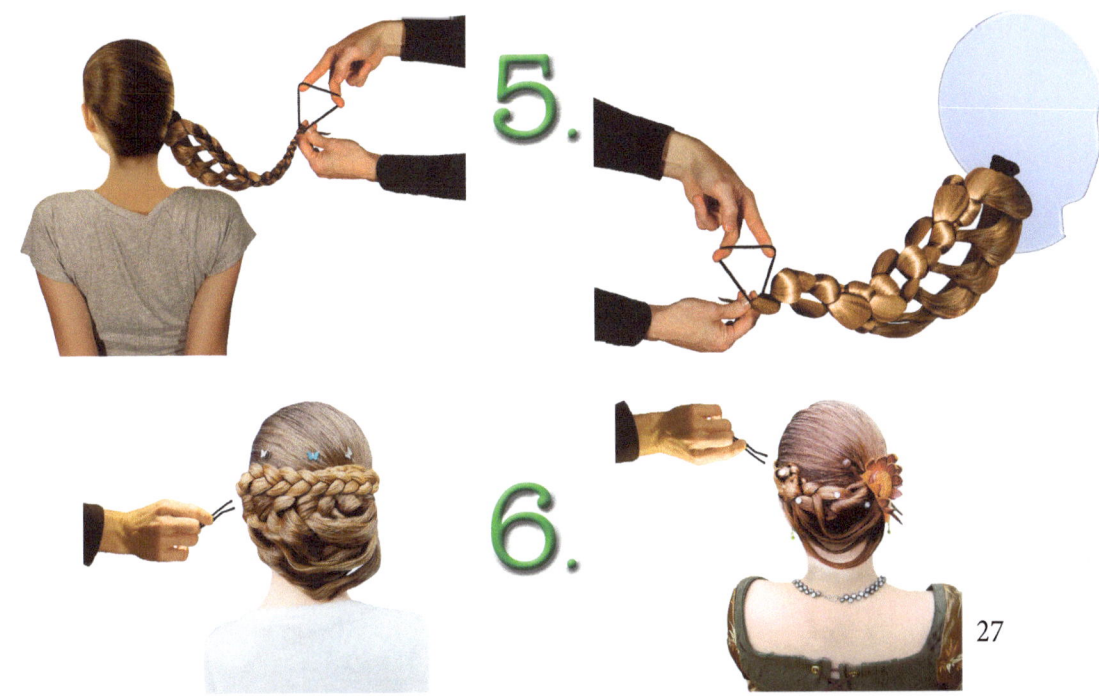

5.

6.

Review

What is a Basic Tail?

When you create a basic tail you make one tail or 100 tails. It doesn't matter where you place the braids as long as all of the hair is used.

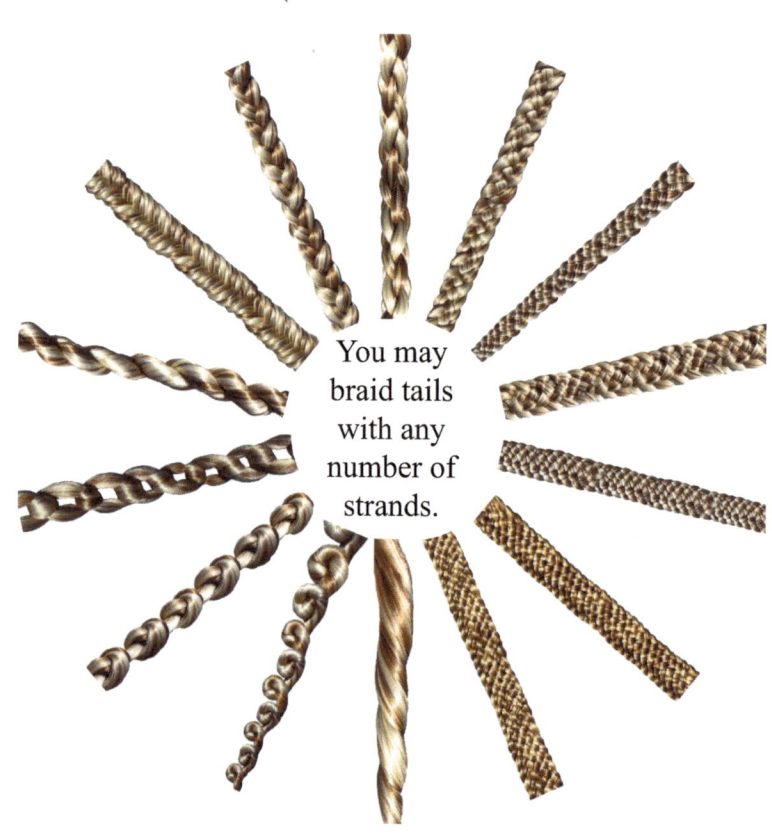

You may braid tails with any number of strands.

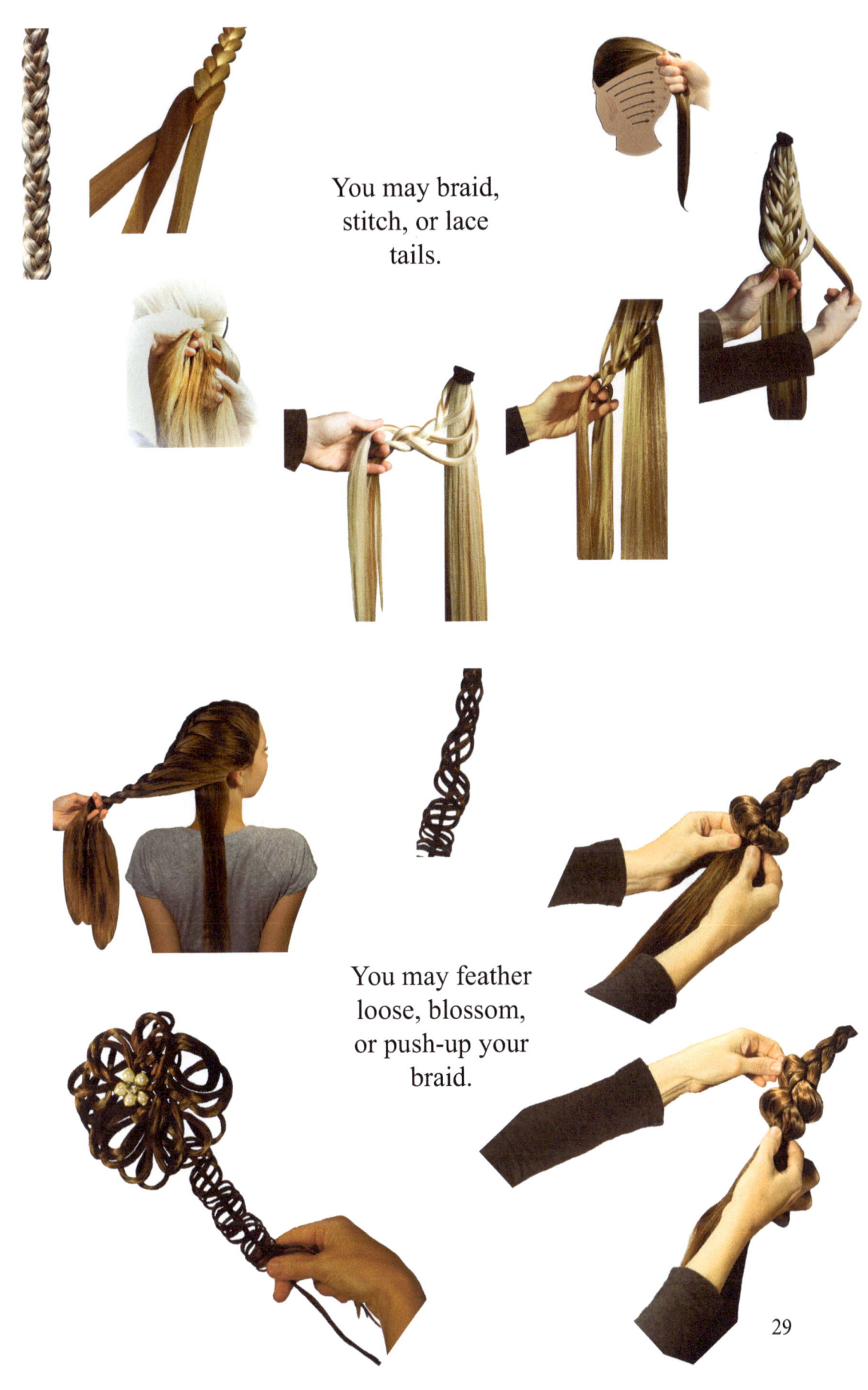

You may braid, stitch, or lace tails.

You may feather loose, blossom, or push-up your braid.

29

Examples

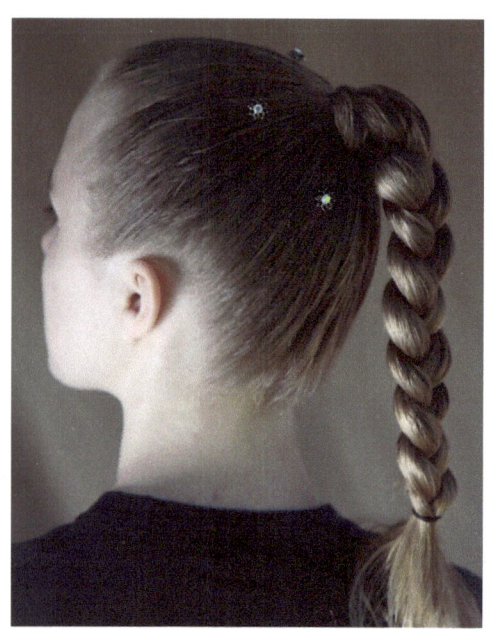
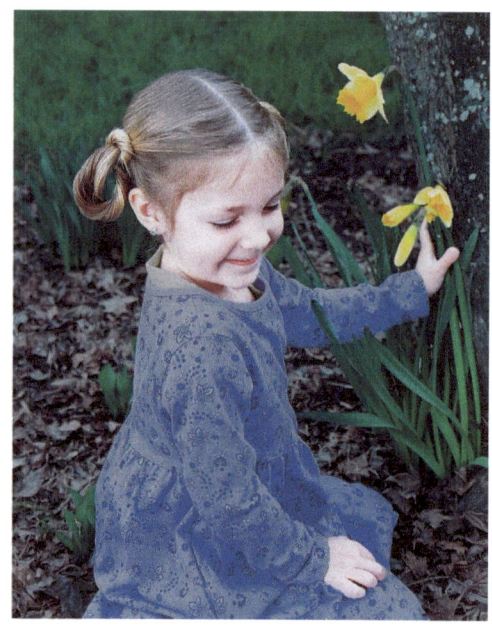
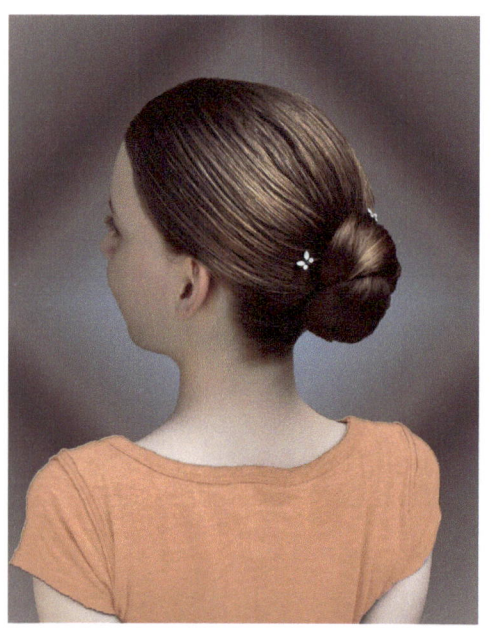
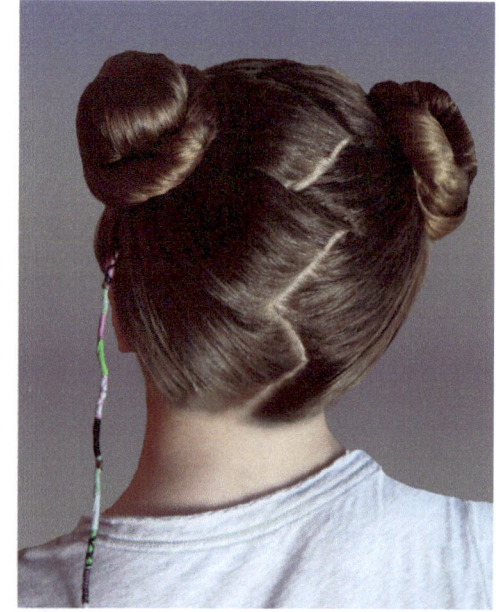

Examples

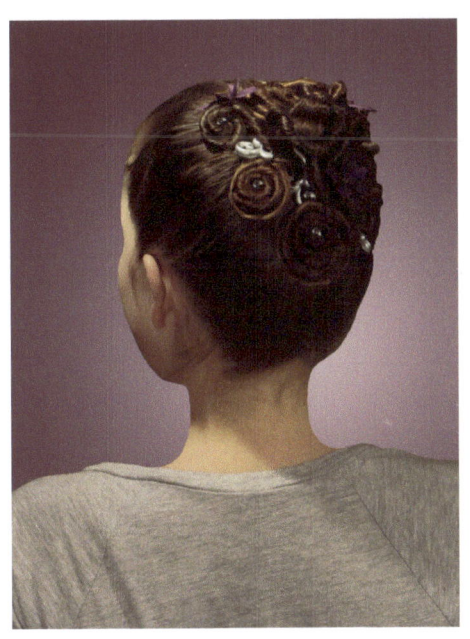 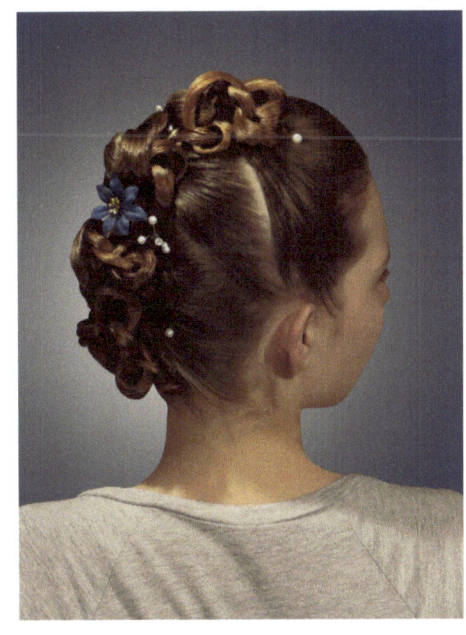

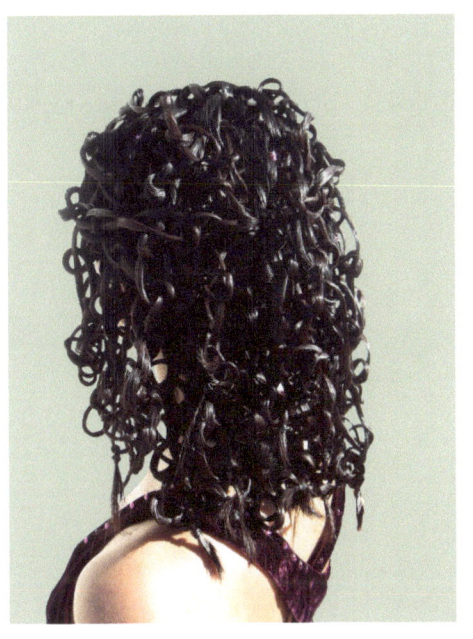 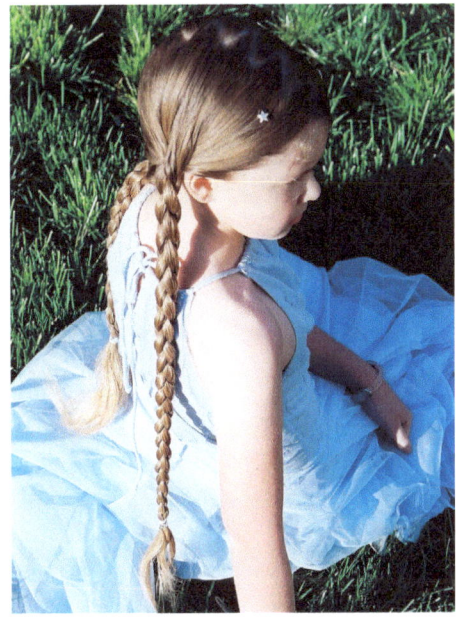

Accented Tails

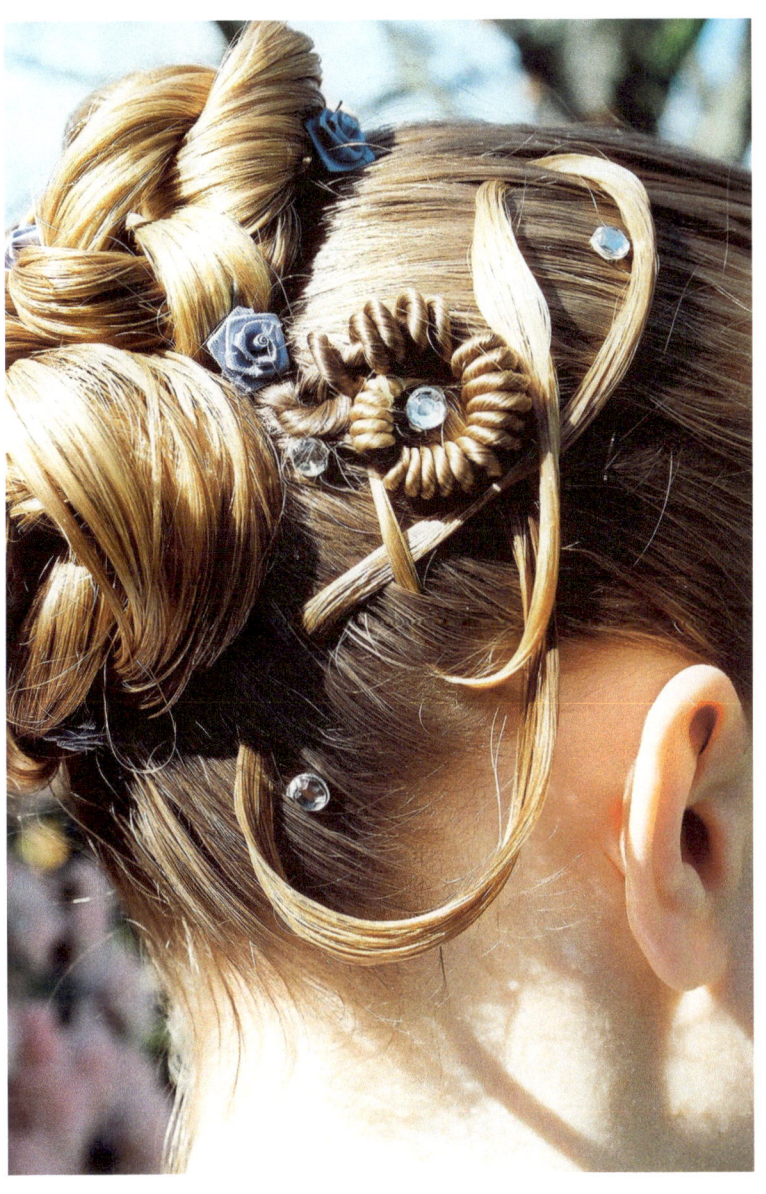

Accent Placements

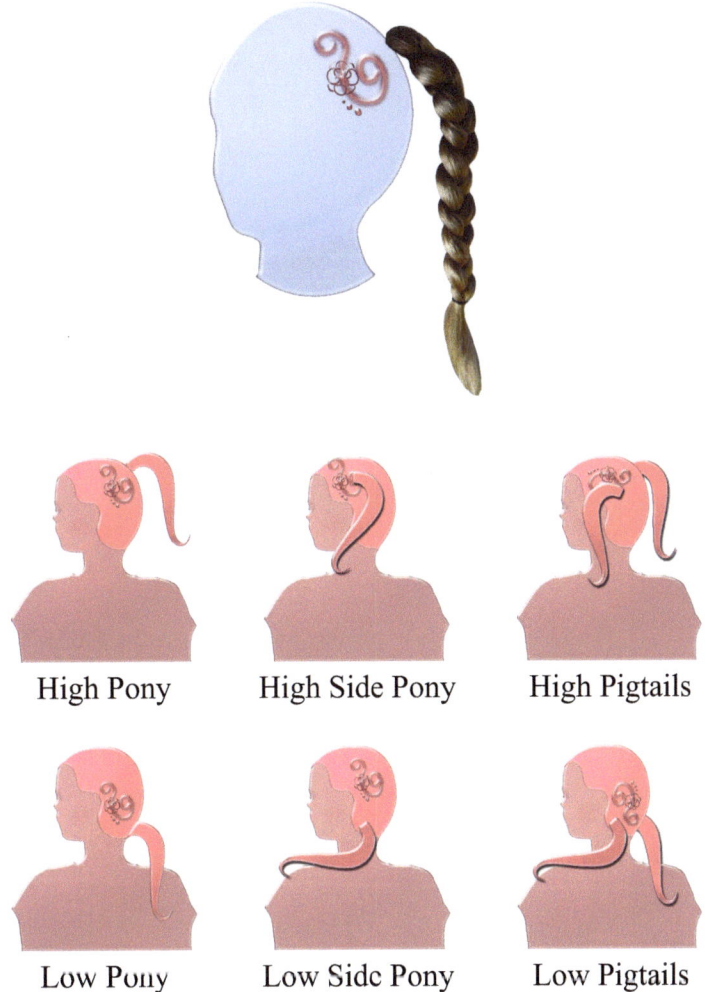

High Pony	High Side Pony	High Pigtails
Low Pony	Low Side Pony	Low Pigtails

The Icons above are suggestions of a few common placements for a tail with accents. As we saw in the previous section there are other placements that I do not show. This is still true in this section for the same reasons. I will make this a small book and I will let you use your imagination and creativity to come up with the other placements, braids, and accents. I can only show so much in this tiny book. I am merely trying to spark your imagination. Try each number of strands that can be braided, with each placement, in combination with each accent possibility. This should keep you busy for years.

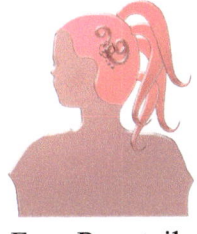

Four Ponytails

Accented

Make one tail or make 100 tails. It doesn't matter where you place the braids as long as all of the hair is used. One or several slivers of hair are left out to create accents. Accents add a decorative flare to any hairstyle including just a plain old unbraided ponytail.

1.

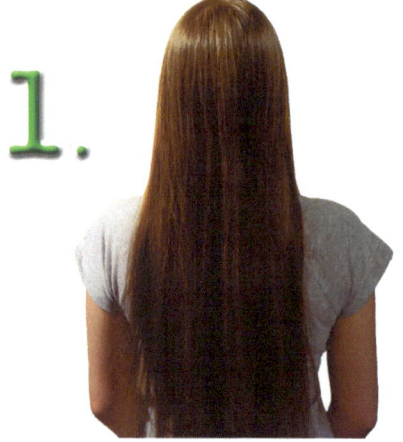

Begin with clean, brushed hair.

2.

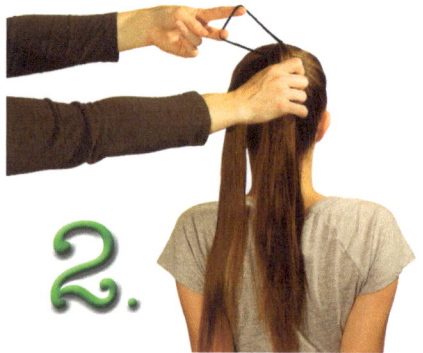

Use a covered rubber band to place most of the hair into a ponytail. I am placing one High Ponytail while leaving out accent hair.

All the examples below are Accented High Ponytails with the ponytails left unbraided.

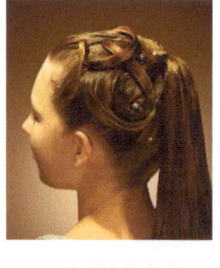
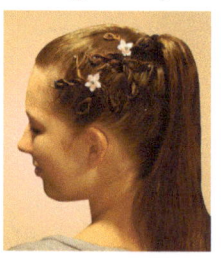
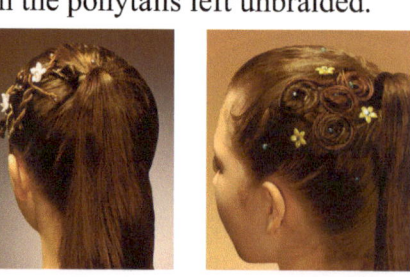

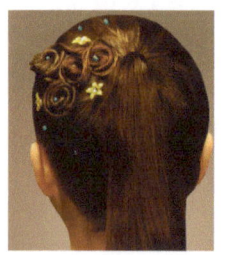
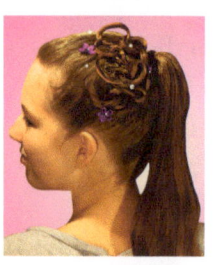
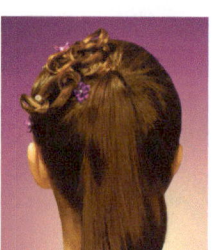
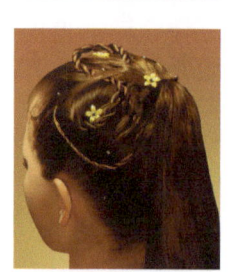
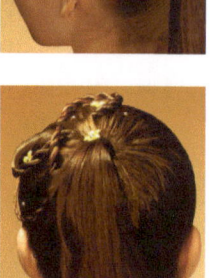

Would you open any of these with a feather loose or blossom?

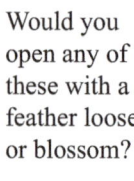
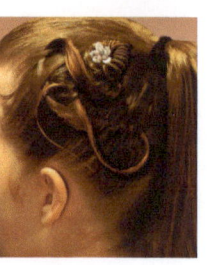
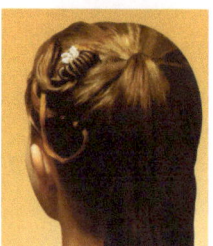
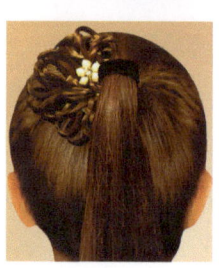
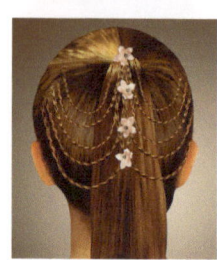

Accented

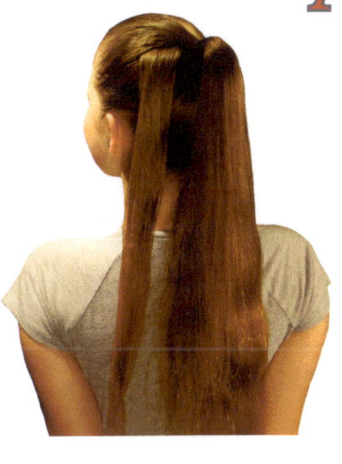

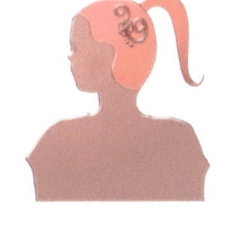

3.

Once you have your accent strands taken out, you will need to decide what the end result will look like.

Will you braid the ponytail? If so, with how many strands, how many braids, and will they hang down or be pinned up?

What accent will be used and how many of them will you be making?

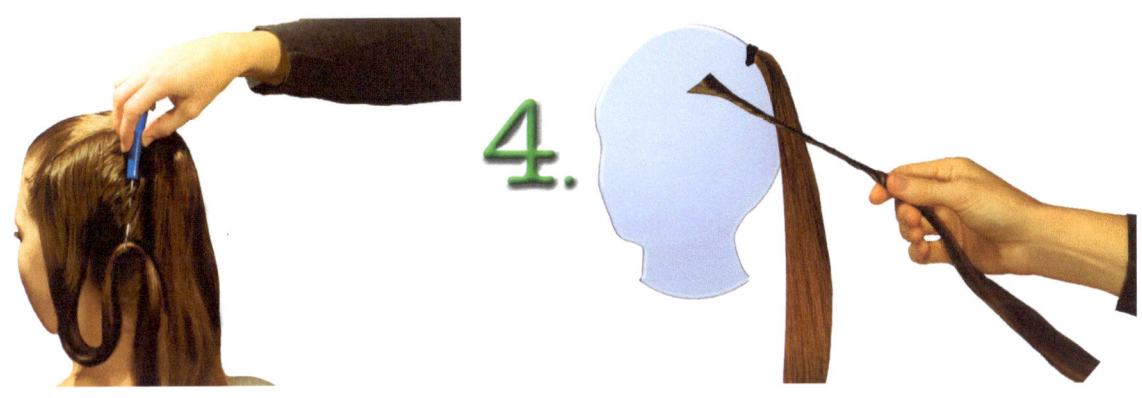

4.

Decide if the accents will hang down or be pinned up.

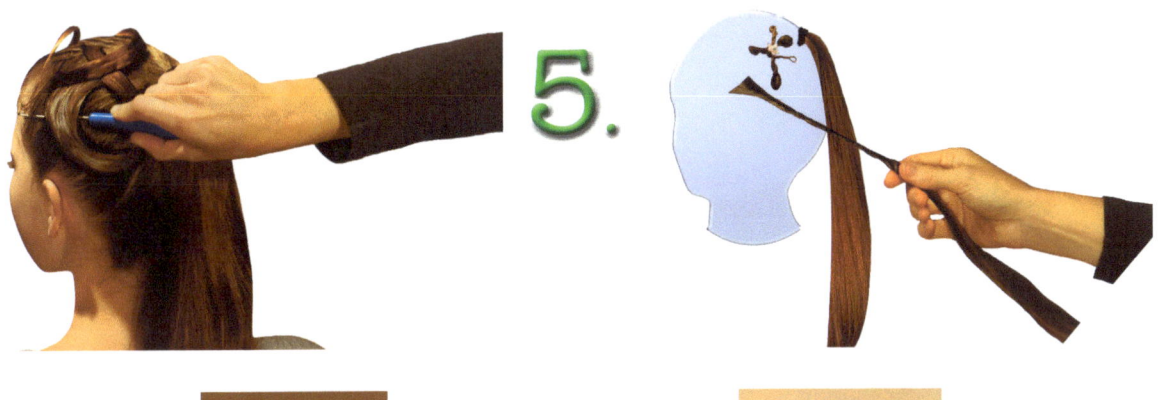

5.

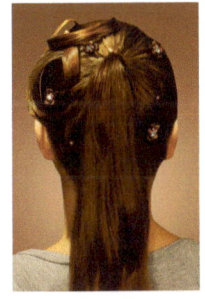

6.

Don't be afraid, these are just ponytails.

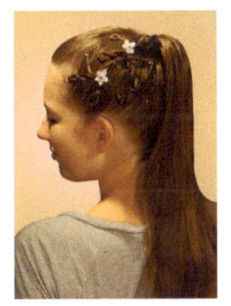

37

Accented

Make one tail or make 100 tails. It doesn't matter where you place the braids as long as all of the hair is used. One or several slivers of hair are left out to create accents. Accents add a decorative flare to any hairstyle including just a plain old unbraided ponytail.

1.

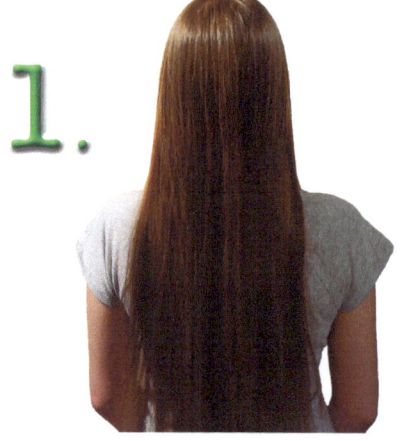

Begin with clean, brushed hair.

2.

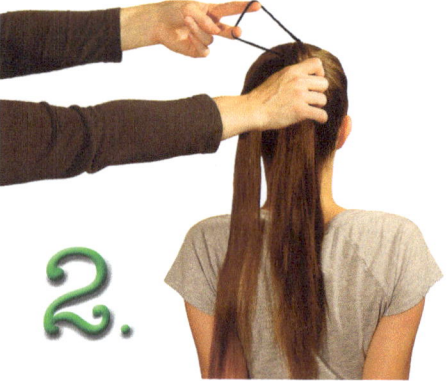

Use a covered rubber band to place most of the hair into a ponytail. I am placing one High Ponytail while leaving out accent hair.

All the examples below are Accented High Ponytails. Some are the ponytails braided, some are the braids pinned up into buns, and some are multiple braids from the ponytail.

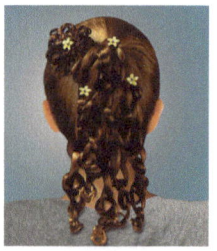
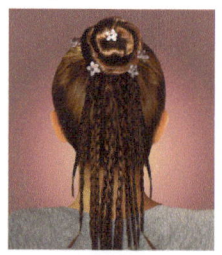
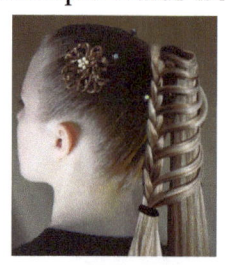
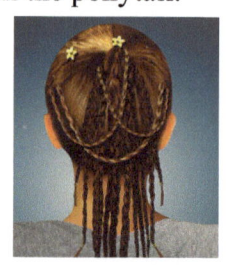

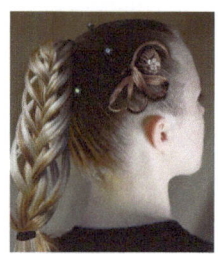
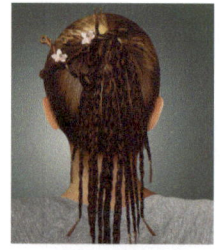
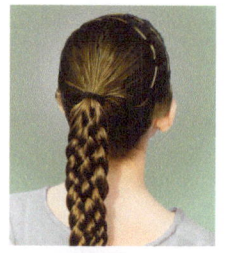
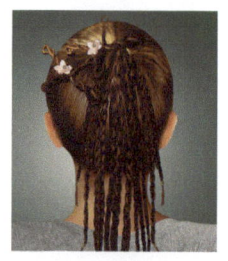
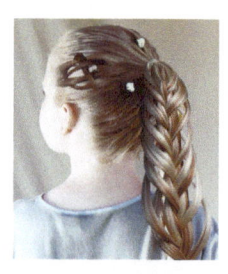

Would you open any of these with a feather loose or blossom?

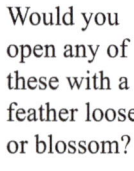
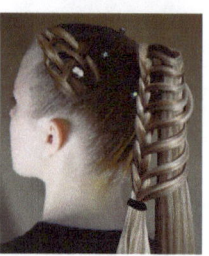
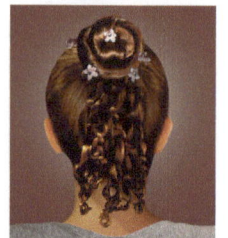
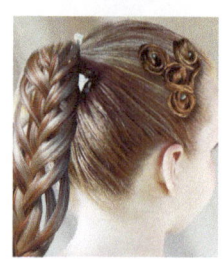
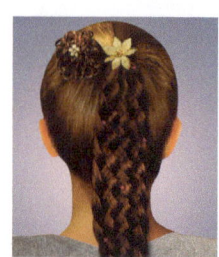

38

Accented

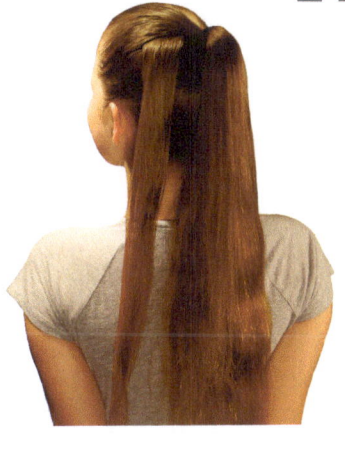

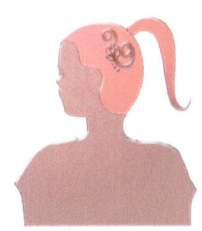

3. Once you have your accent strands taken out, you will need to decide what the end result will look like.

Will you braid the ponytail? If so, with how many strands and how many braids? Will they hang down or be pinned up?

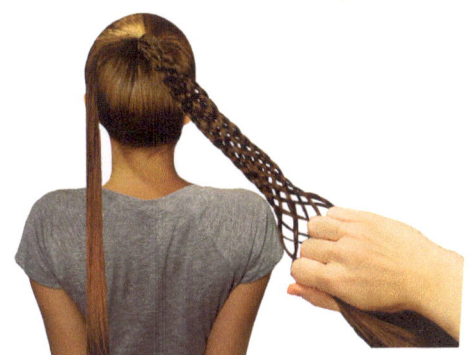

4.

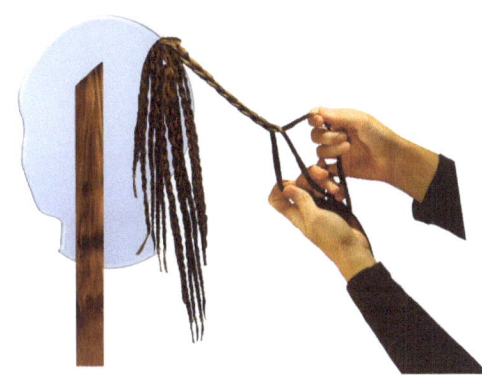

What accent will be used and how many of them will you be making?

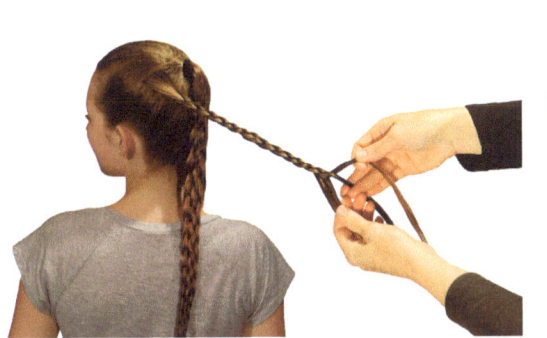

5.

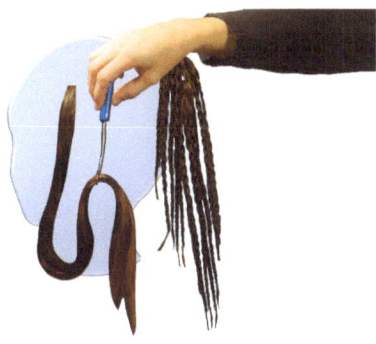

Decide if the accents will hang down or be pinned up.

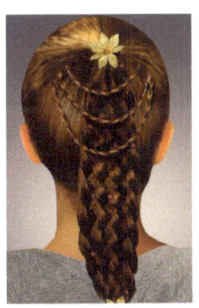

6.

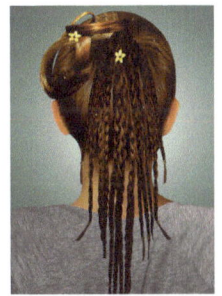

39

Accented

Make one tail or make 100 tails. It doesn't matter where you place the braids as long as all of the hair is used. One or several slivers of hair are left out to create accents. Accents add a decorative flare to any hairstyle including just a plain old unbraided ponytail.

1.

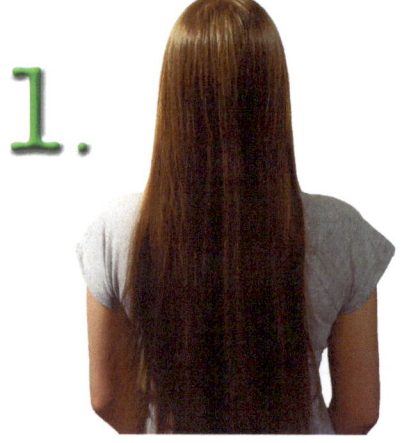

Begin with clean, brushed hair.

2.

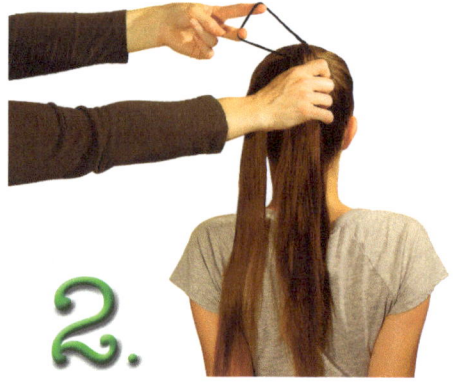

Use a covered rubber band to place most of the hair into a ponytail. I am placing one High Ponytail while leaving out accent hair.

All the examples below are Accented High Ponytails. All are pinned up into buns, some are multiple braids pinned up.

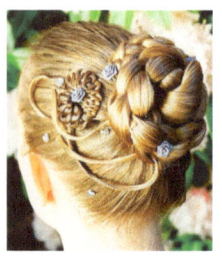
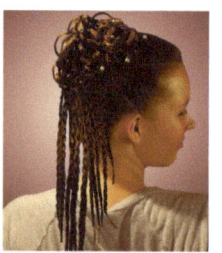
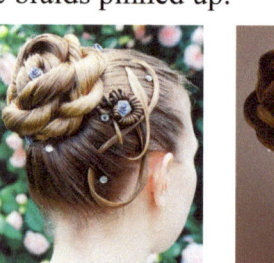
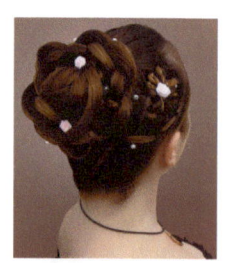

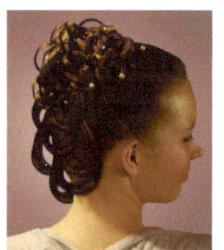
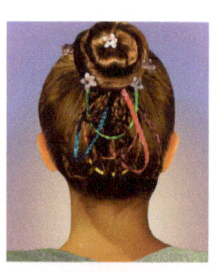
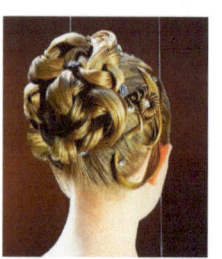
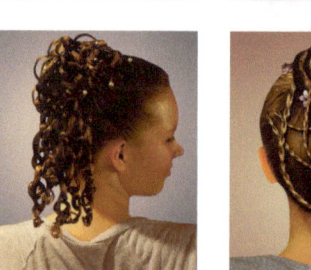

Would you open any of these with a feather loose or blossom?

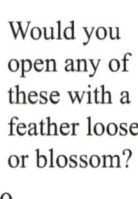
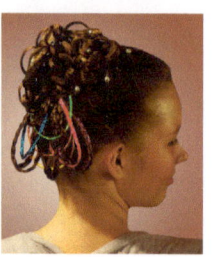
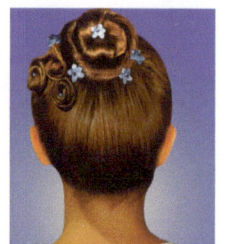
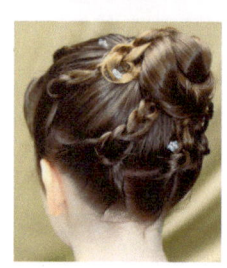
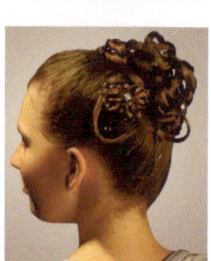

40

Accented

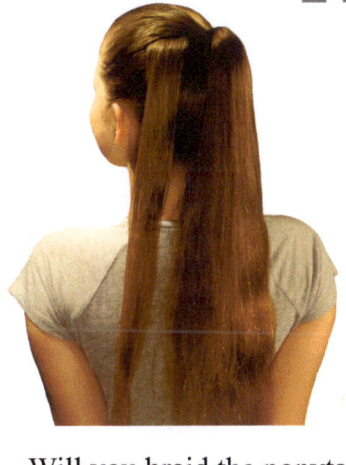

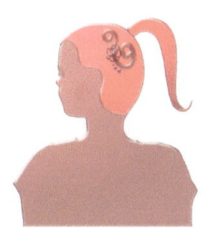

3. Once you have your accent strands taken out, you will need to decide what the end result will look like.

Will you braid the ponytail? If so, with how many strands and how many braids? Will they hang down or be pinned up?

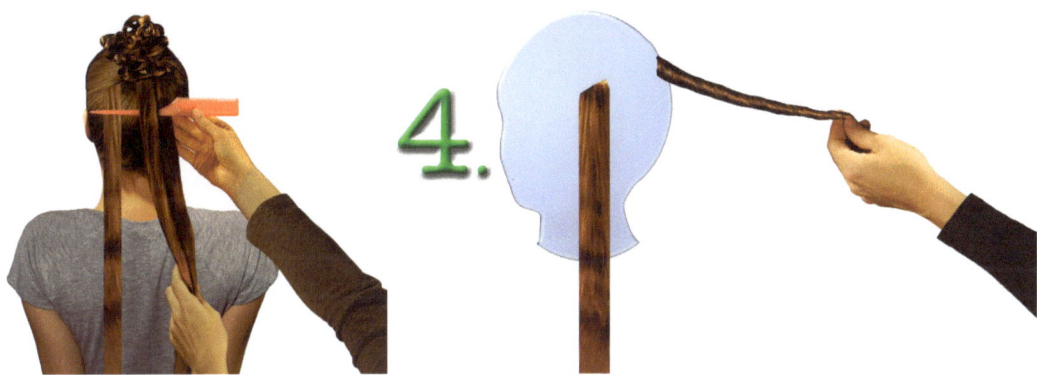

4.

What accent will be used and how many of them will you be making?

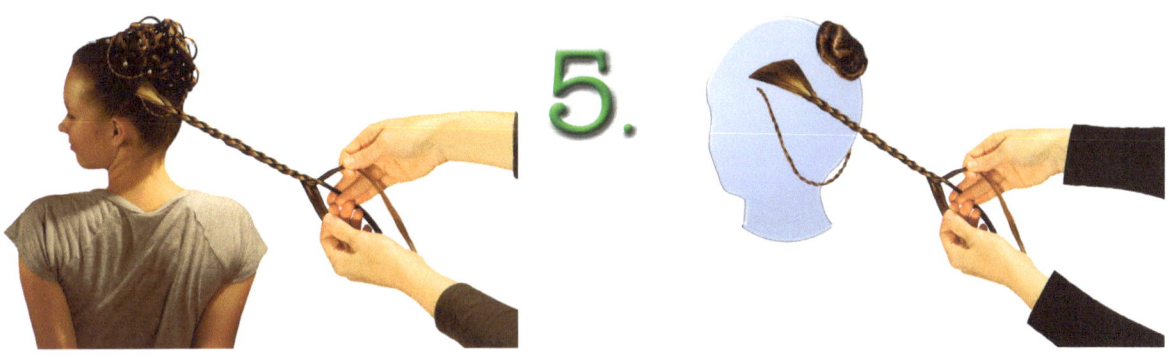

5.

Decide if the accents will hang down or be pinned up.

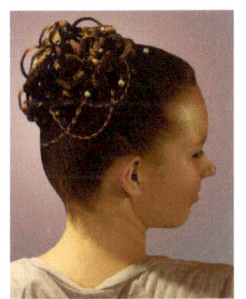

6.

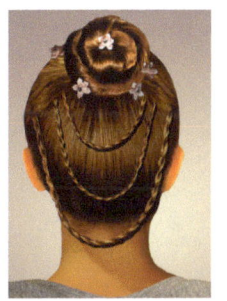

Accented

Make one tail or make 100 tails. It doesn't matter where you place the braids as long as all of the hair is used. One or several slivers of hair are left out to create accents. Accents add a decorative flare to any hairstyle including just a plain old unbraided ponytail.

1.

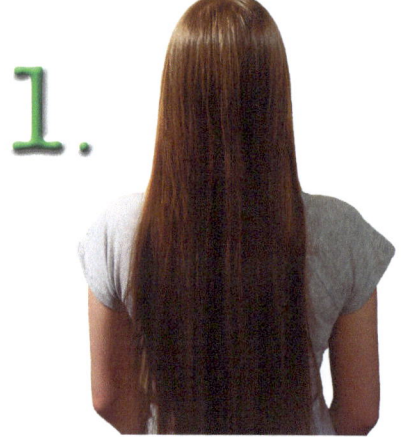

Begin with clean, brushed hair.

2.

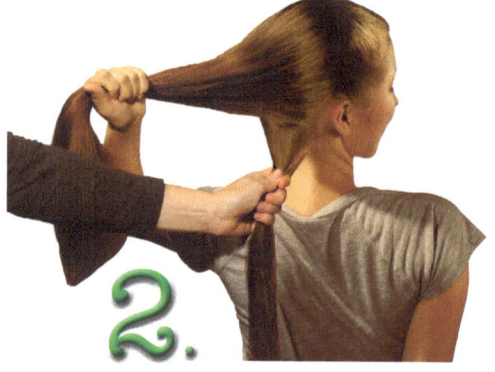

Use a covered rubber band to place most of the hair into a ponytail. I am placing one Low Ponytail while leaving out accent hair.

All the examples below are Accented Low Ponytails. All are pinned up into buns, some are multiple braids pinned up.

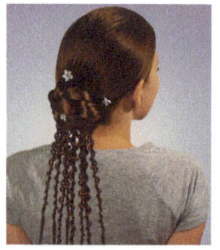
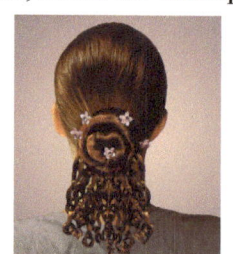
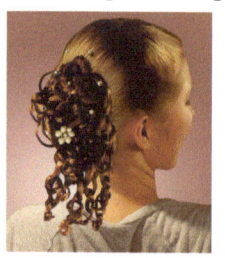
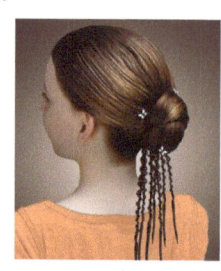

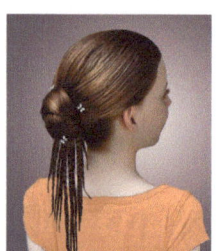
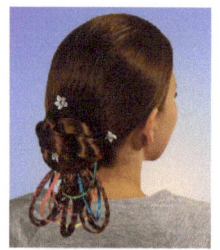
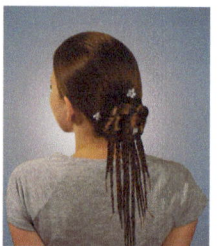
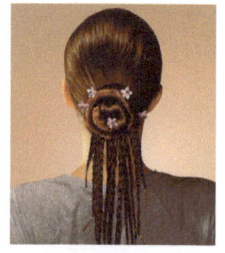
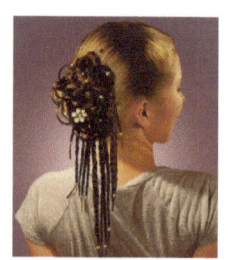

Would you open any of these with a feather loose or blossom?

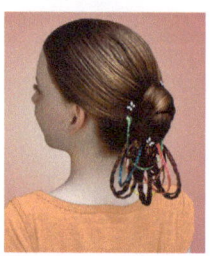
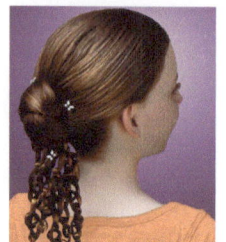
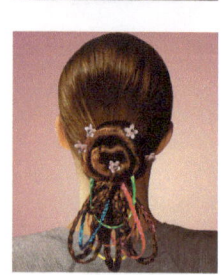
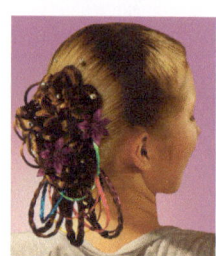

Accented

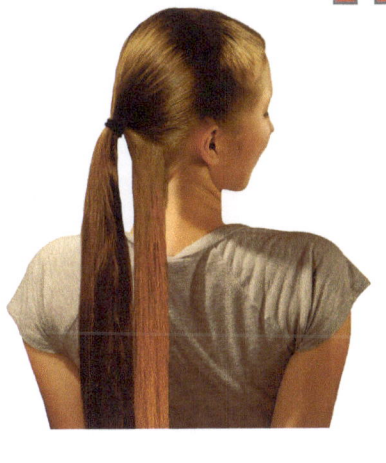

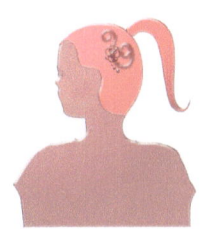

3. Once you have your accent strands taken out, you will need to decide what the end result will look like.

Will you braid the ponytail? If so, with how many strands and how many braids? Will they hang down or be pinned up?

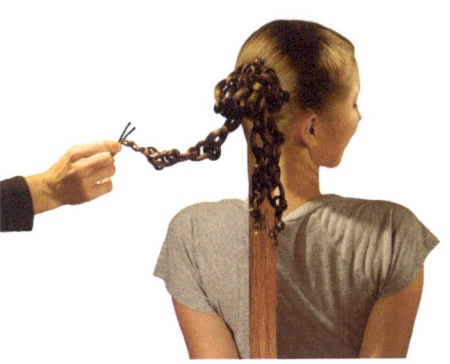

4.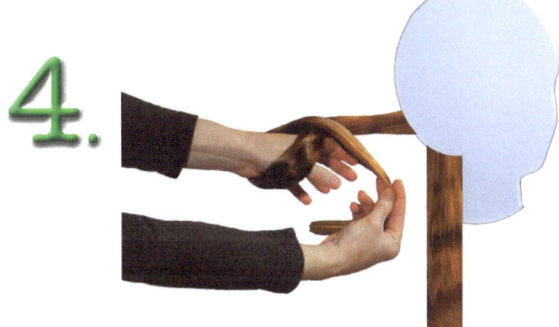

What accent will be used and how many of them will you be making?

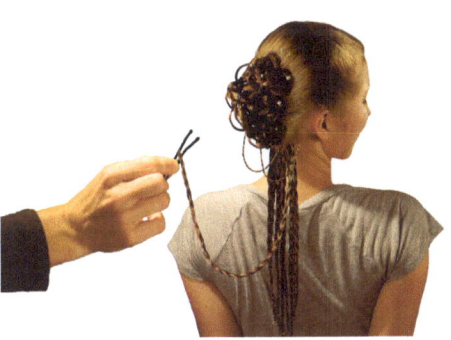

5.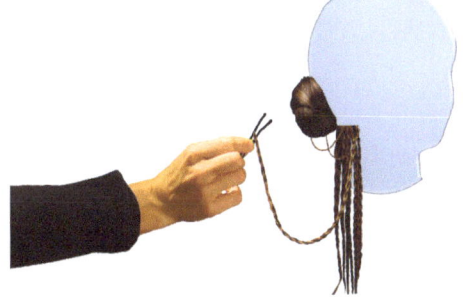

Decide if the accents will hang down or be pinned up.

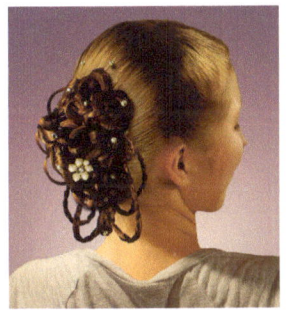

6.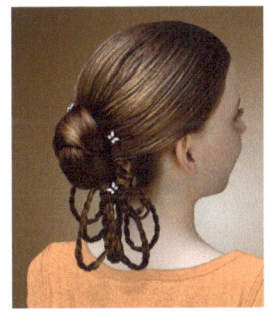

Accented

Make one tail or make 100 tails. It doesn't matter where you place the braids as long as all of the hair is used. One or several slivers of hair are left out to create accents. Accents add a decorative flare to any hairstyle including just a plain old unbraided ponytail.

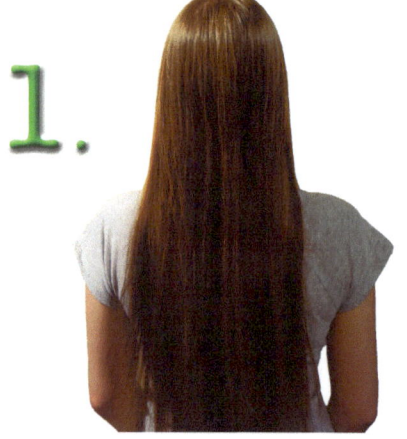

1.

Begin with clean, brushed hair.

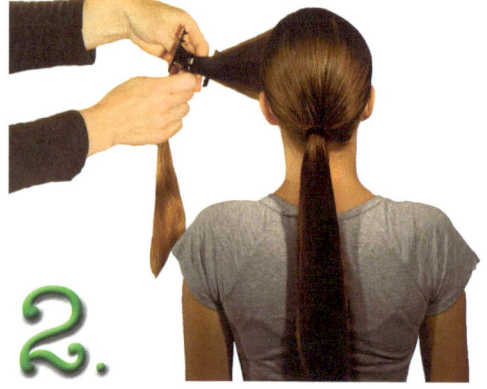

2.

Use a covered rubber band to place most of the hair into a ponytail. I am placing one Low Ponytail while leaving out accent hair.

All the examples below are Accented Low Ponytails. Some are the ponytails braided and some are multiple braids from the ponytail.

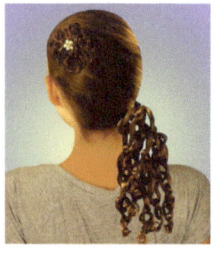
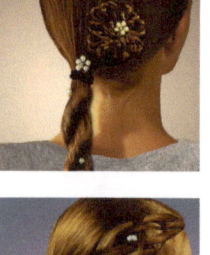
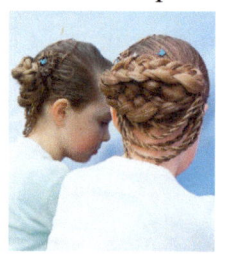
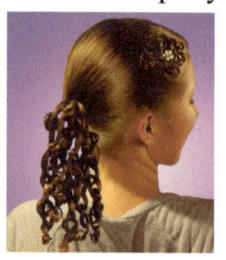
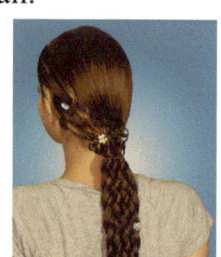

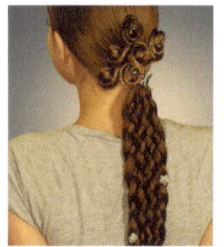
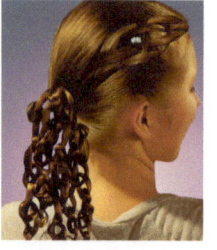
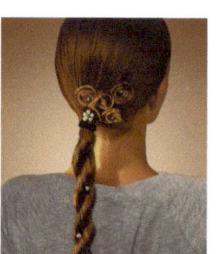
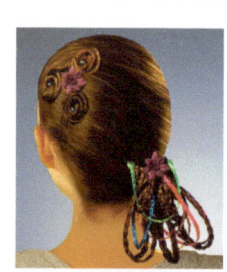
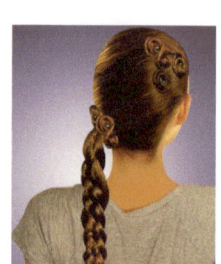

Would you open any of these with a feather loose or blossom?

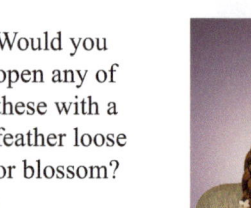
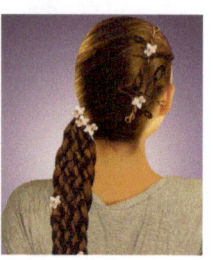
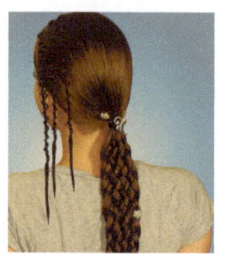
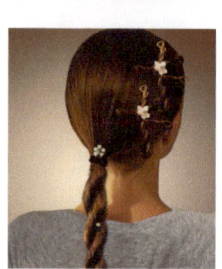
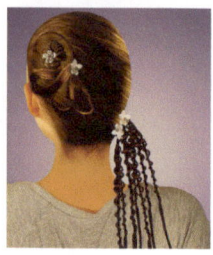

44

Accented

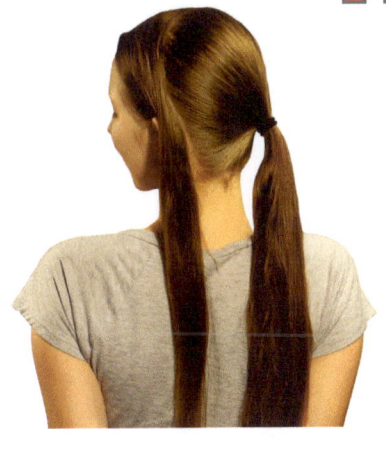
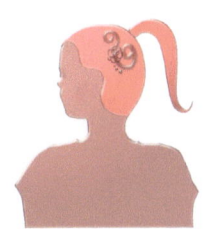

3.

Once you have your accent strands taken out, you will need to decide what the end result will look like.

Will you braid the ponytail? If so, with how many strands and how many braids? Will they hang down or be pinned up?

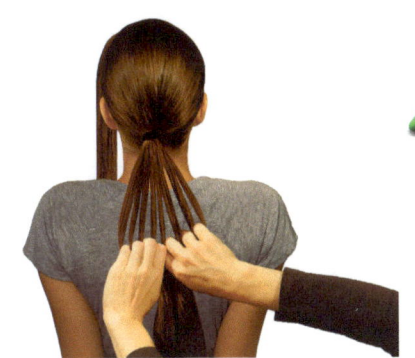

4.

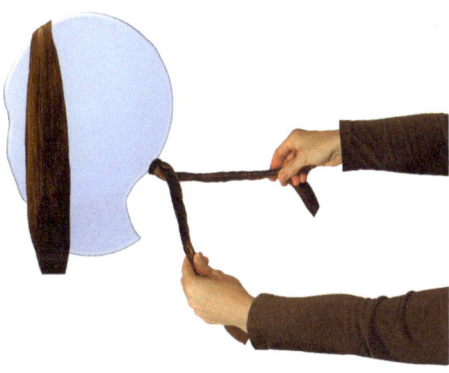

What accent will be used and how many of them will you be making?

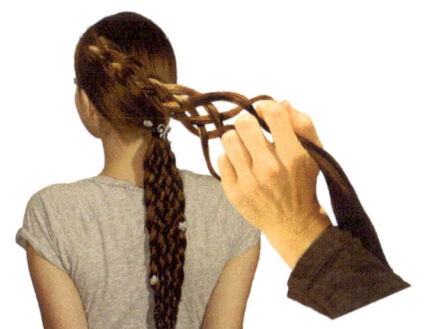

5.

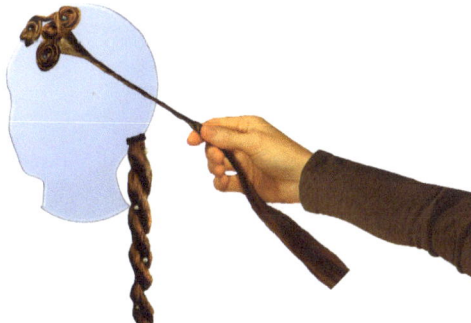

Decide if the accents will hang down or be pinned up.

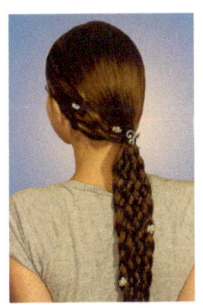

6.

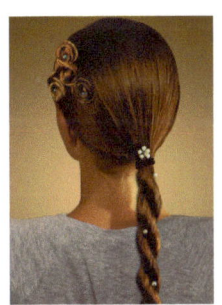

Accented

Make one tail or make 100 tails. It doesn't matter where you place the braids as long as all of the hair is used. One or several slivers of hair are left out to create accents. Accents add a decorative flare to any hairstyle including just a plain old unbraided ponytail.

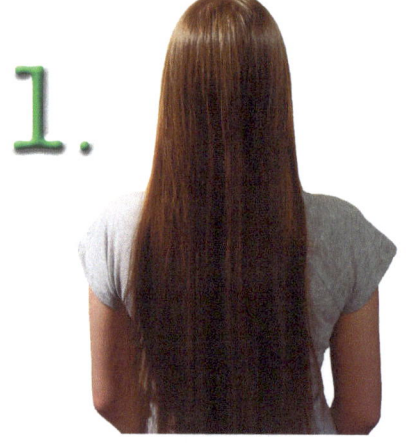

1.

Begin with clean, brushed hair.

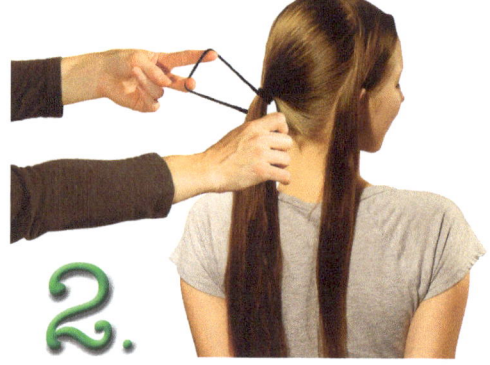

2.

Use a covered rubber band to place most of the hair into a ponytail. I am placing one Low Ponytail while leaving out accent hair.

All the examples below are Accented Low Ponytails. All are pinned up into buns, some are multiple braids pinned up.

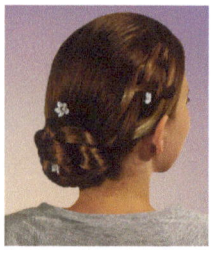
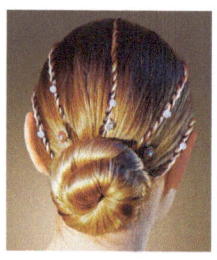
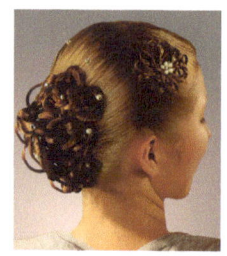
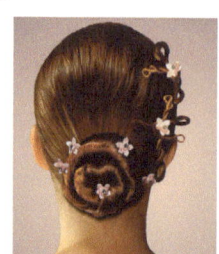

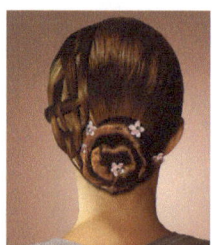
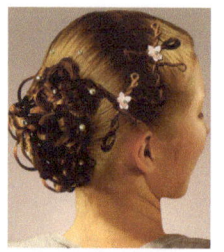
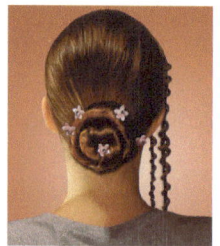
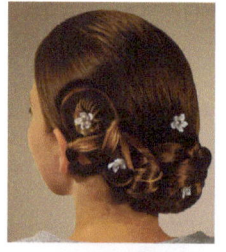
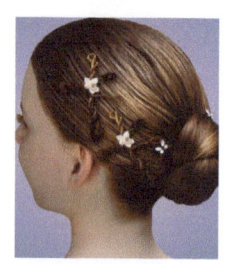

Would you open any of these with a feather loose or blossom?

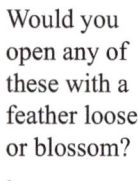
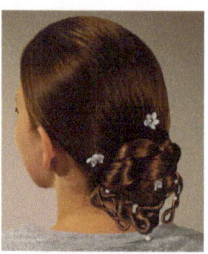
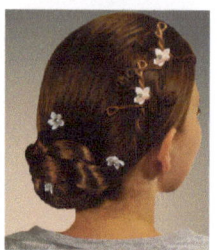
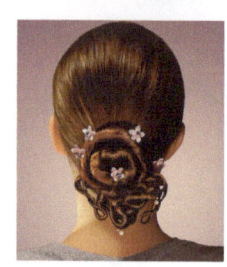
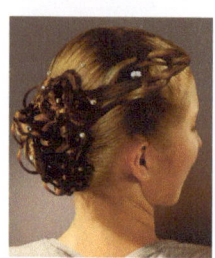

Accented

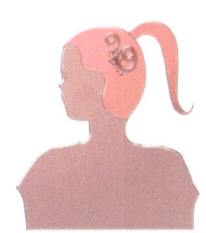

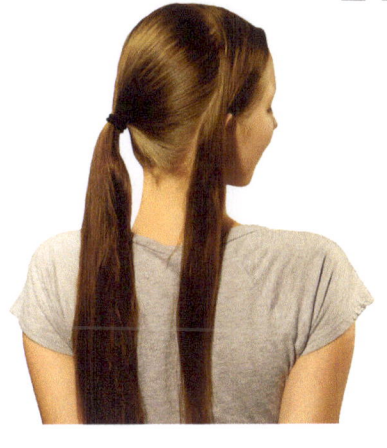

3. Once you have your accent strands taken out, you will need to decide what the end result will look like.

Will you braid the ponytail? If so, with how many strands and how many braids? Will they hang down or be pinned up?

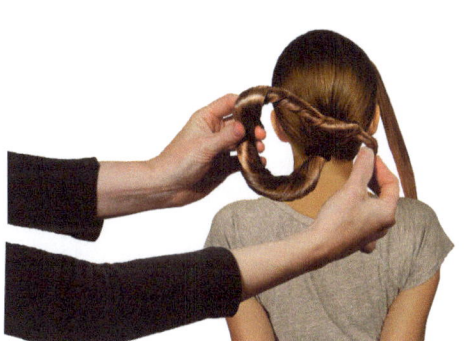

4.

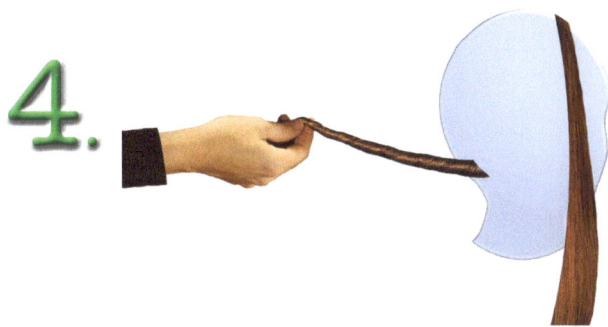

What accent will be used and how many of them will you be making?

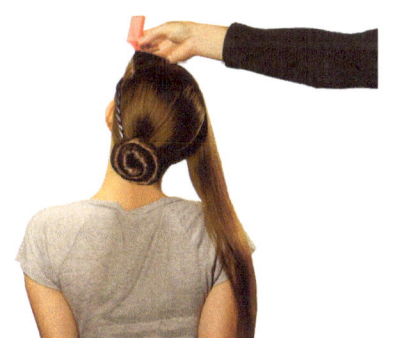

5.

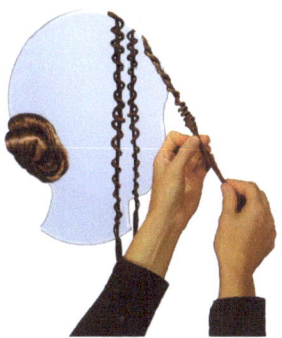

Decide if the accents will hang down or be pinned up.

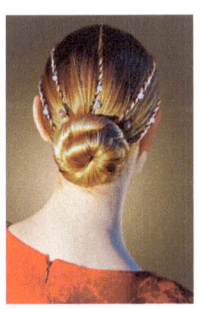

6.

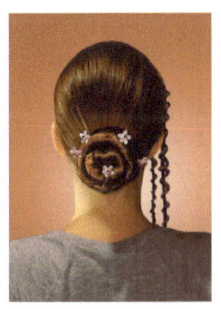

Review

What is an Accented Tail?

When you create an accented tail you make one tail or 100 tails. It doesn't matter where the braids are placed as long as all of the hair is used. One or several slivers of hair are left out to create accents. Accents add a decorative flare to any hairstyle including just a plain old unbraided ponytail.

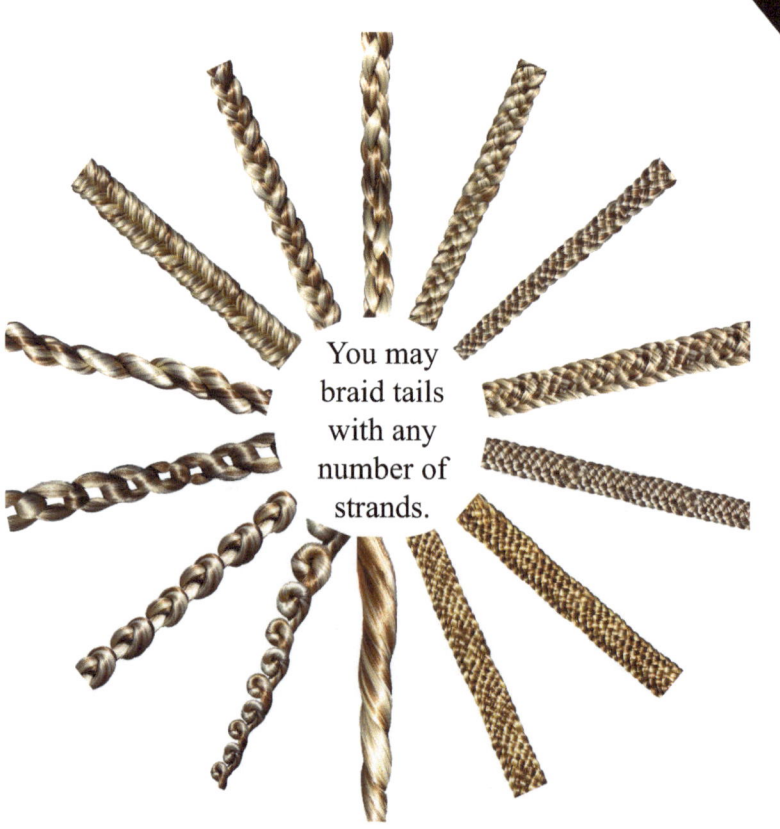

You may braid tails with any number of strands.

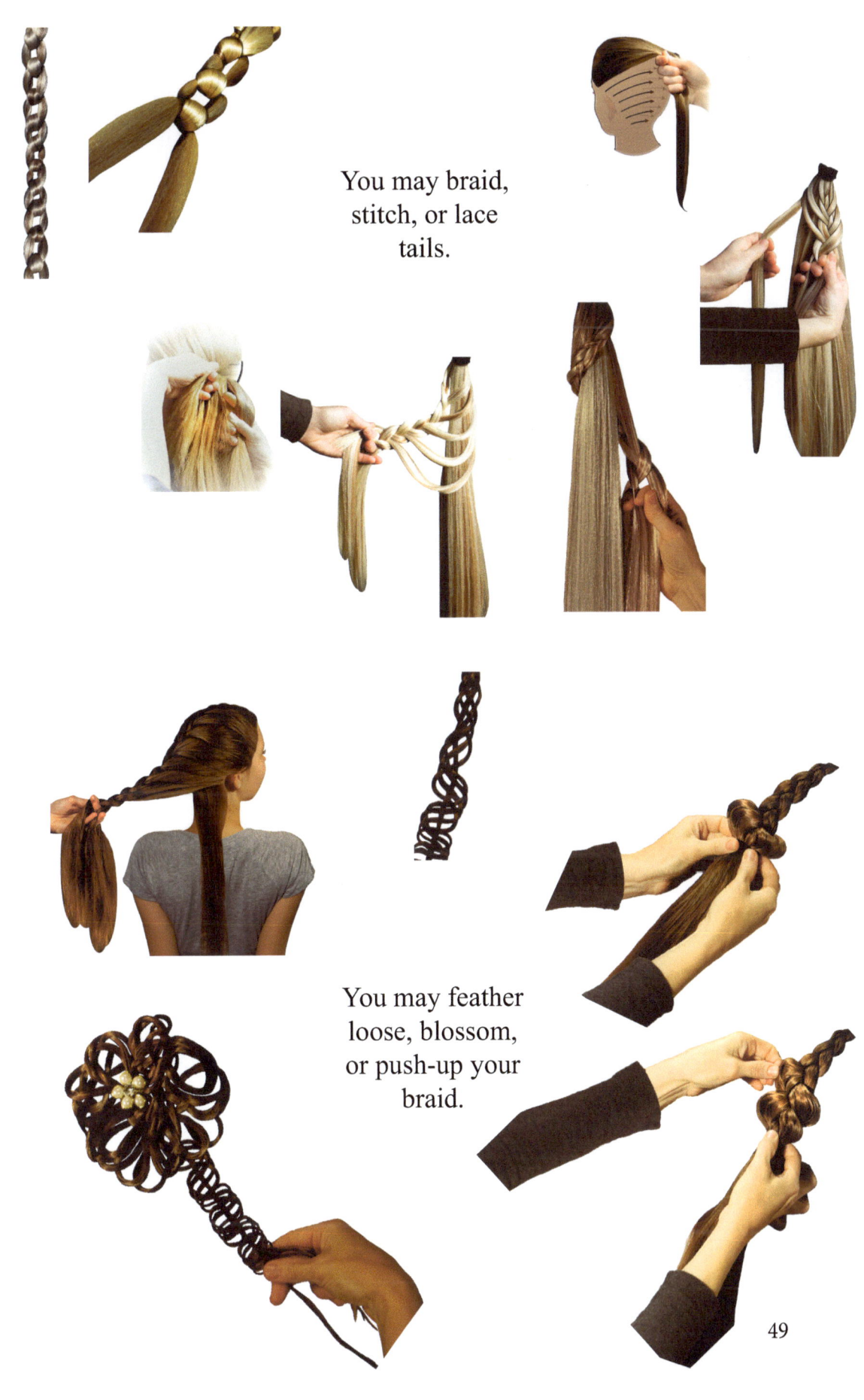

You may braid,
stitch, or lace
tails.

You may feather
loose, blossom,
or push-up your
braid.

49

Examples

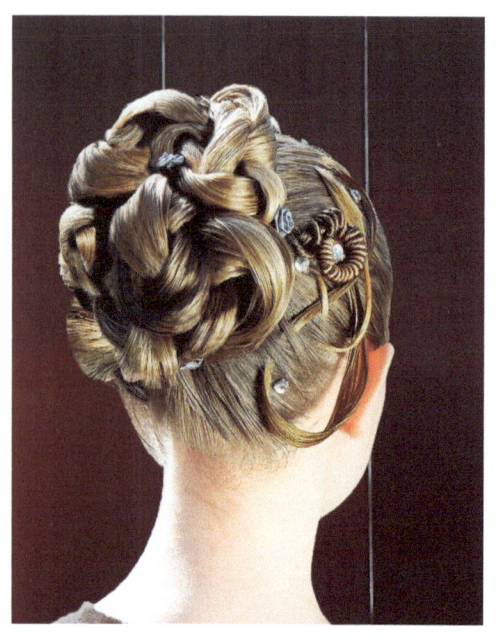
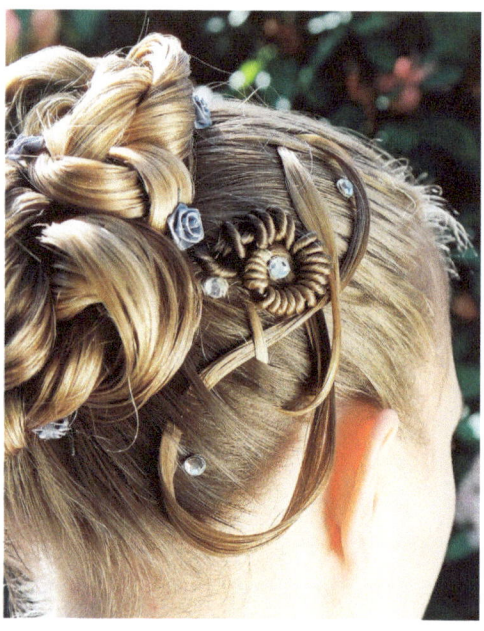
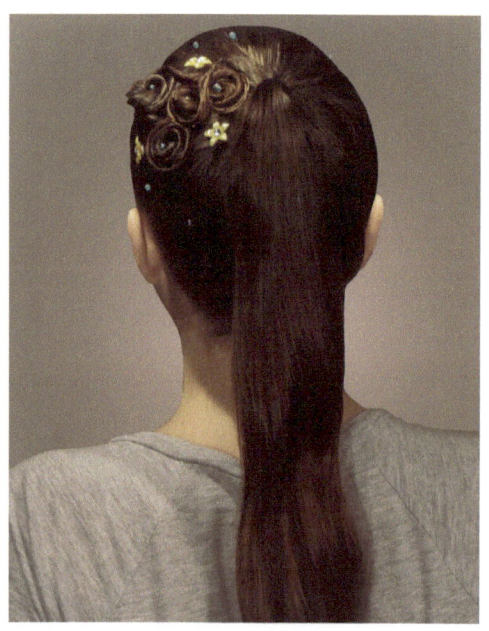
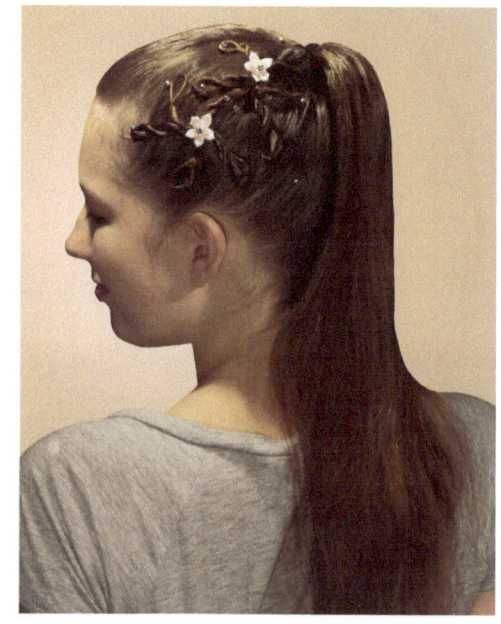

Examples

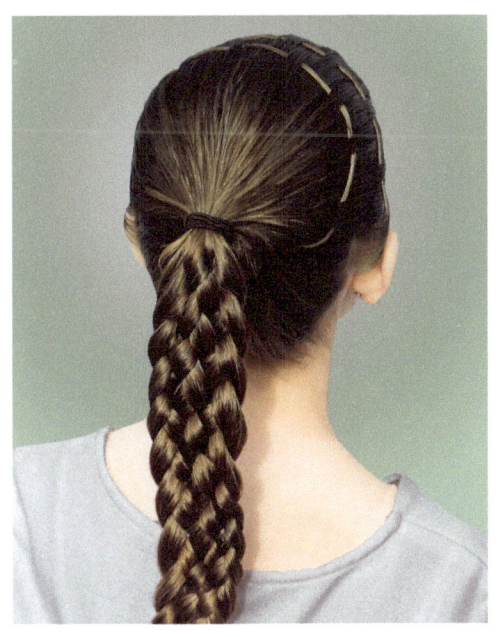
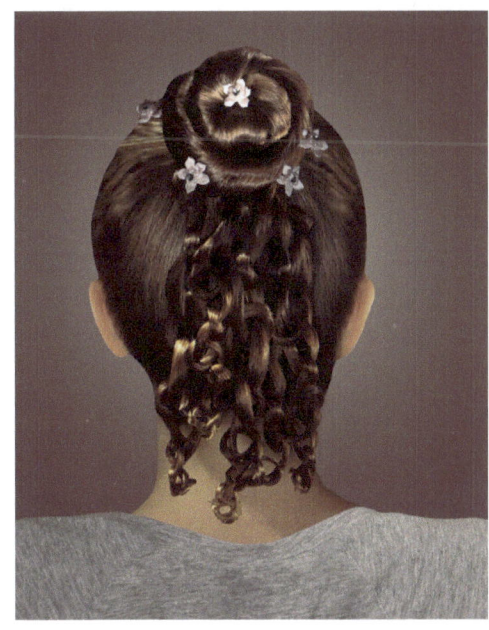
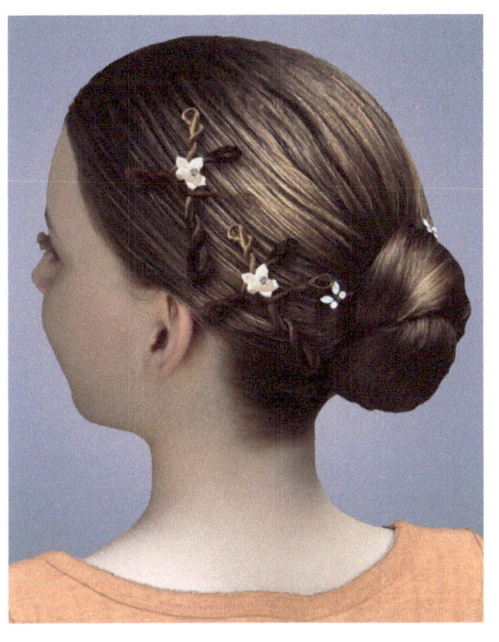
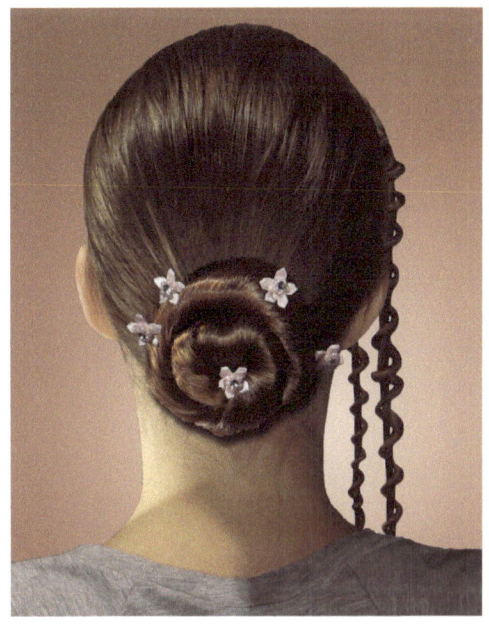

Cascade
Tails

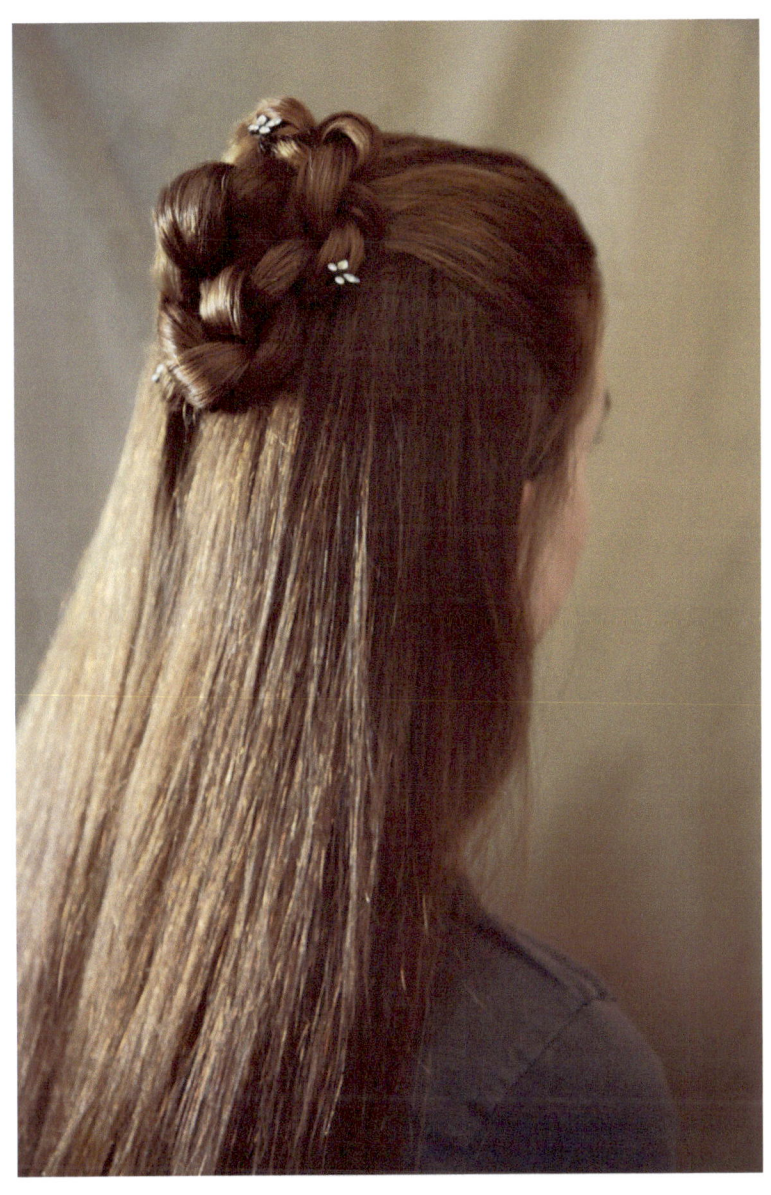

Cascade Placement

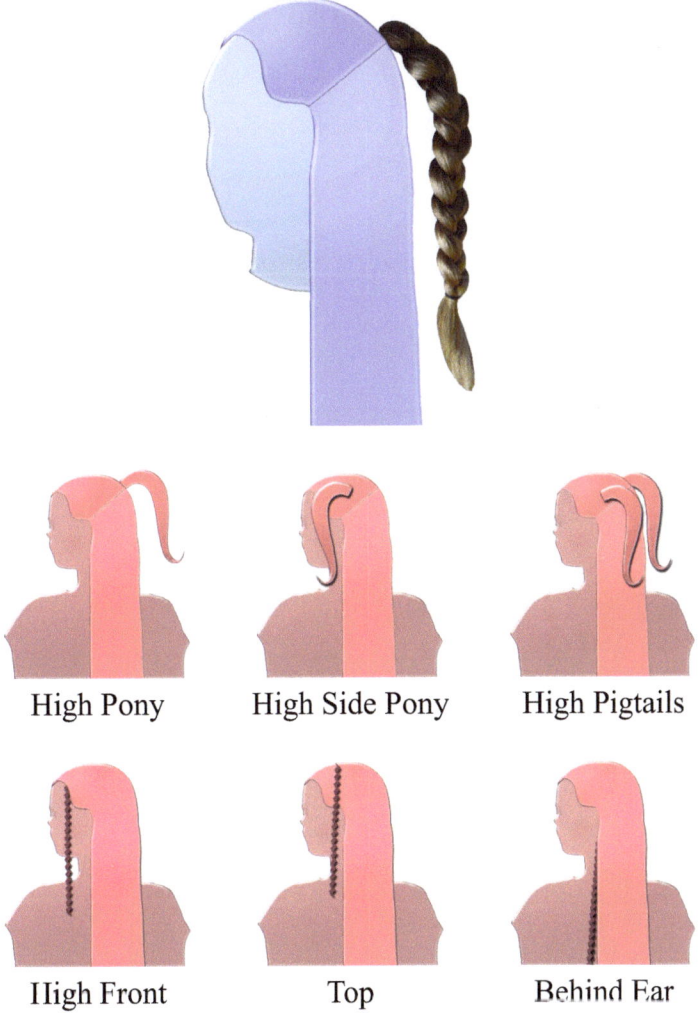

High Pony   High Side Pony   High Pigtails

High Front   Top   Behind Ear

The Icons above are suggestions of a few common placements for the cascade. How many placements can you think of that I have not suggested? Can you imagine how thick this book would be if I showed each one? I made this a small book so you will need to use your imagination to come up with other placements.

And as always, please refer to previous sections for more ideas. Each example may be modified to fit other sections of the book. If you love a hairstyle from the basic section of he book but wish it had half the hair down, then do that hairstyle leaving half the hair down.

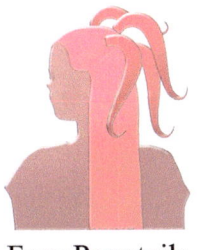

Four Ponytails

Cascade

Make one tail or make 100 tails. It doesn't matter where you place the braids as long as half of the hair is left out.

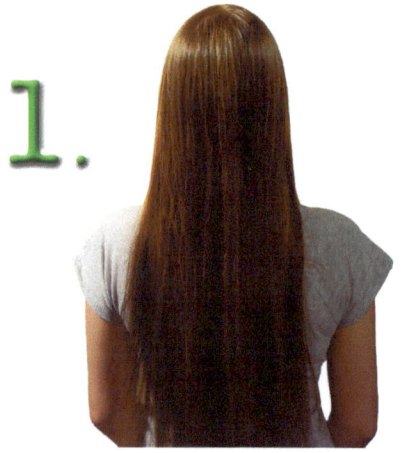

1.

Begin with clean, brushed hair.

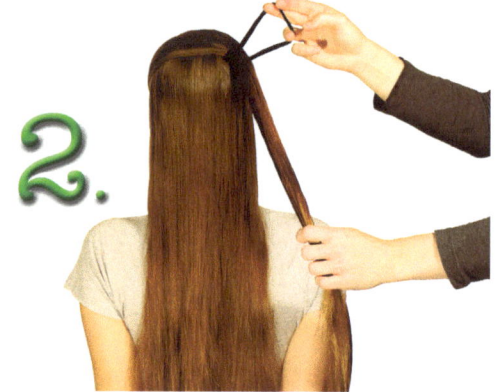

2.

Use a covered rubber band to place part of the hair into a ponytail. Leave out the cascade.

All the examples below have one ponytail. Some are just the tail braided, some are the braids pinned up into buns, and some are multiple braids from the ponytail.

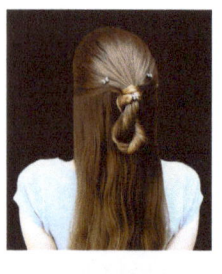
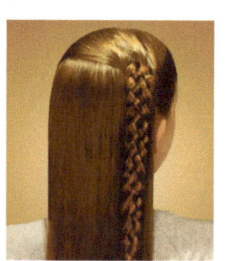
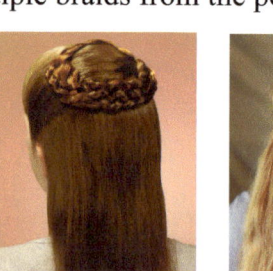
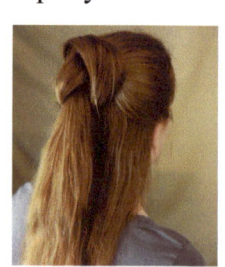

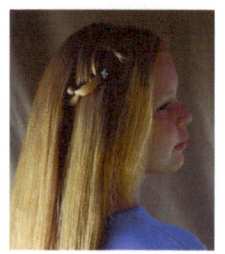
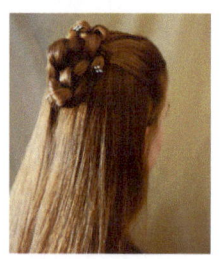
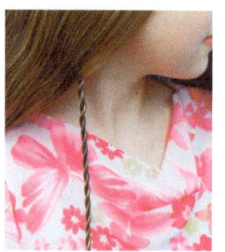
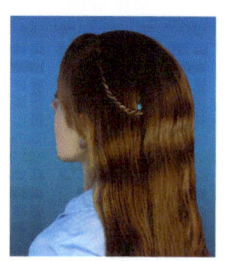
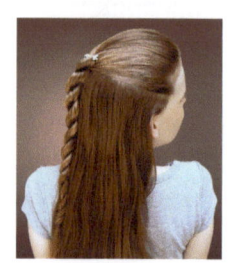

Would you open any of these with a feather loose or blossom?

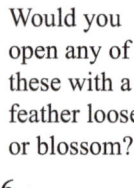
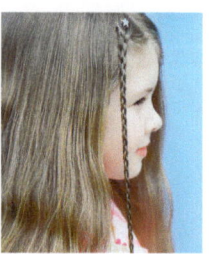
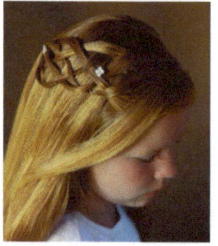
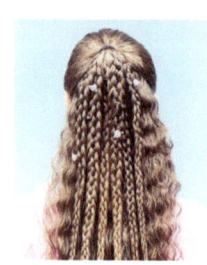
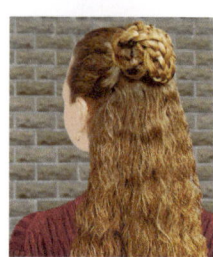

56

Cascade

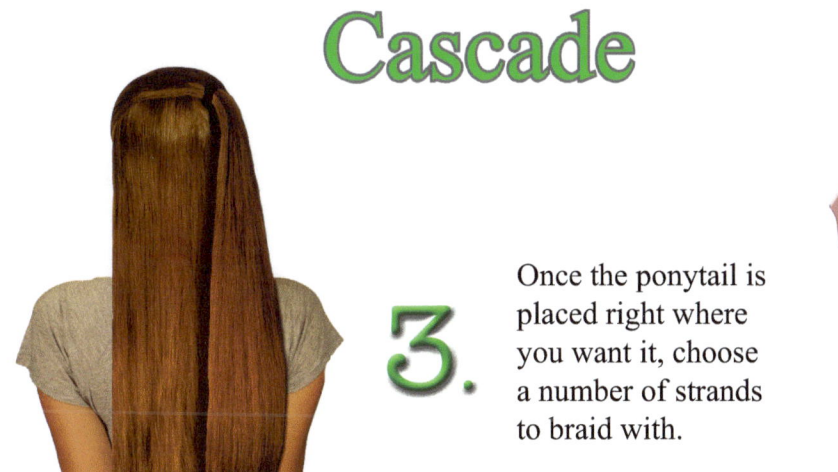

3. Once the ponytail is placed right where you want it, choose a number of strands to braid with.

After the number of strands has been chosen, decide how many braids will be made.

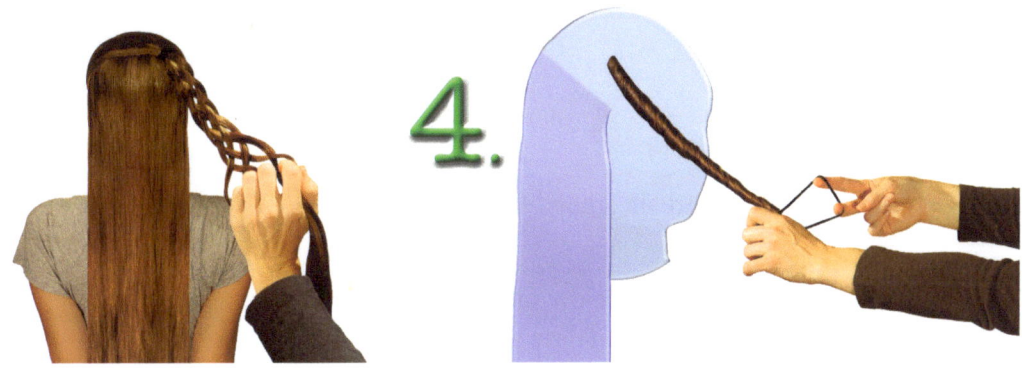

4.

Finally, determine if those braids will hang down or be pinned up.

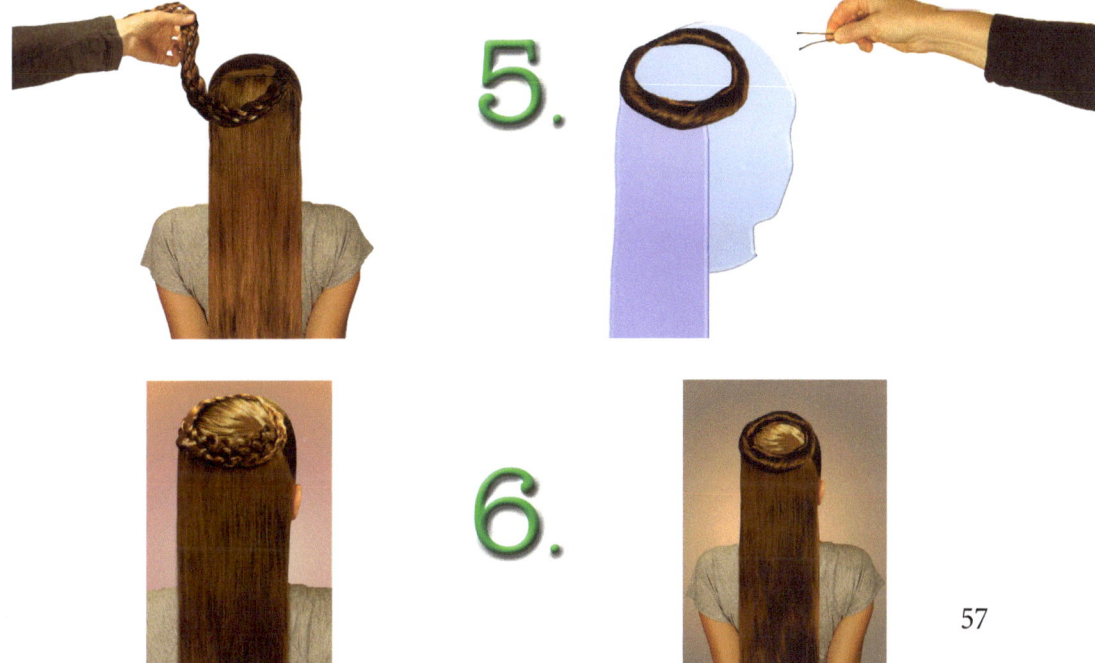

5.

6.

Cascade

Make one tail or make 100 tails. It doesn't matter where you place the braids as long as half of the hair is left out.

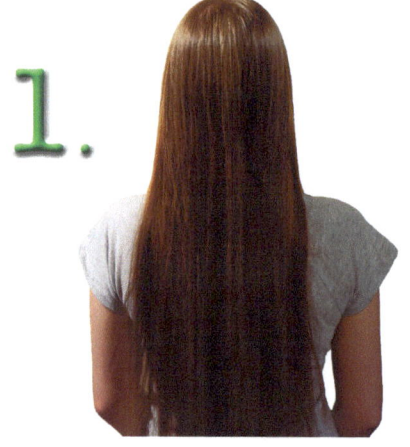

1.

Begin with clean, brushed hair.

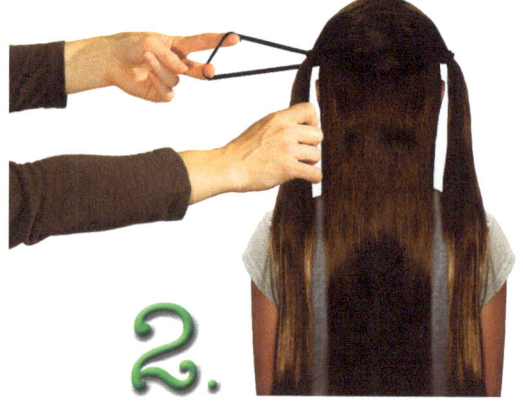

2.

Use covered rubber bands to create two tails. Leave out the cascade.

All the examples below use two tails. Some are just the tails braided, while some are the braids pinned up into buns.

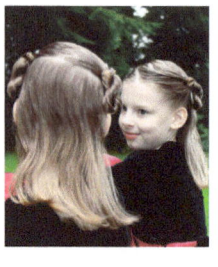
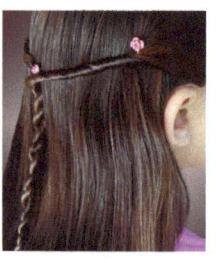
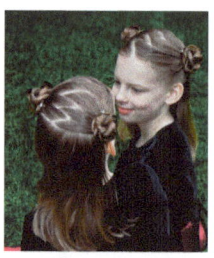
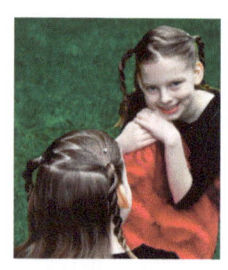
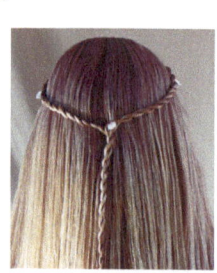

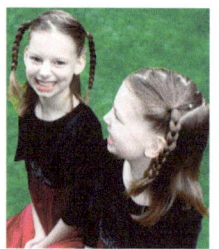
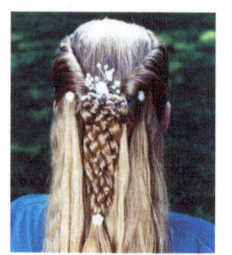
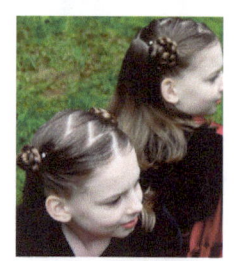
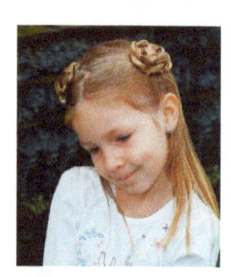

Would you open any of these with a feather loose or blossom?

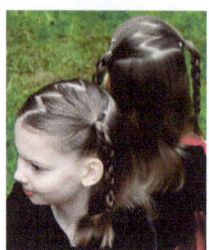
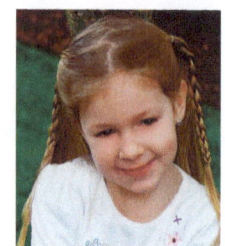
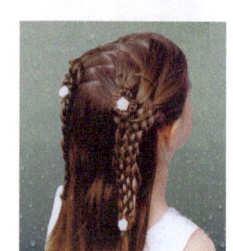
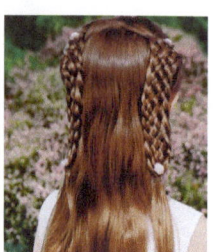

Cascade

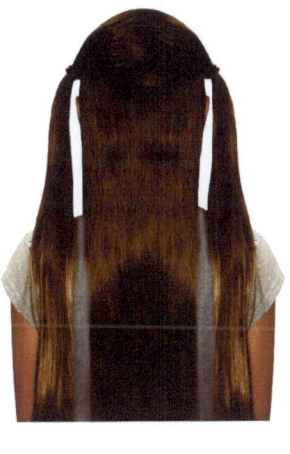

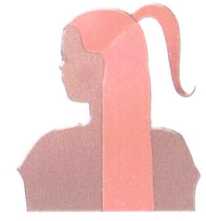

3. Once the ponytails are placed right where you want them, choose a number of strands to braid with.

After the number of strands has been chosen, decide how many braids will be made.

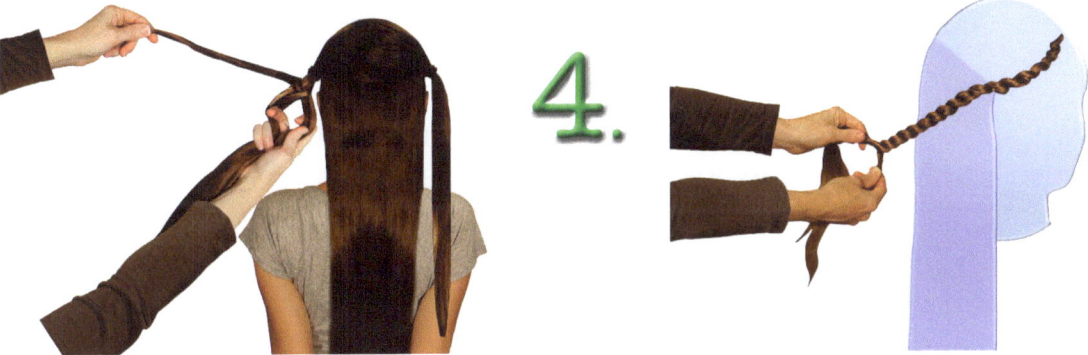

4.

Finally, determine if those braids will hang down or be pinned up.

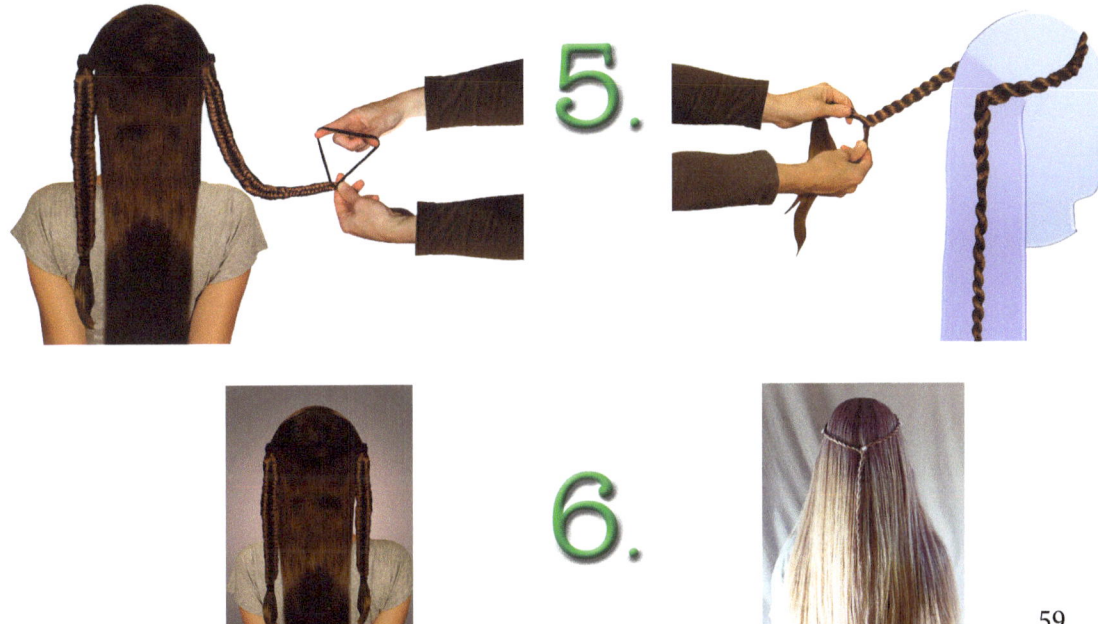

5.

6.

Cascade

Make one tail or make 100 tails. It doesn't matter where you place the braids as long as half of the hair is left out.

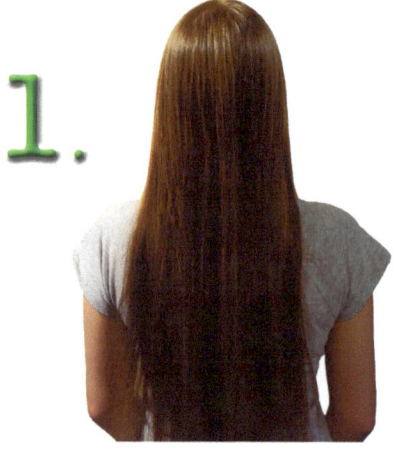

1.

Begin with clean, brushed hair.

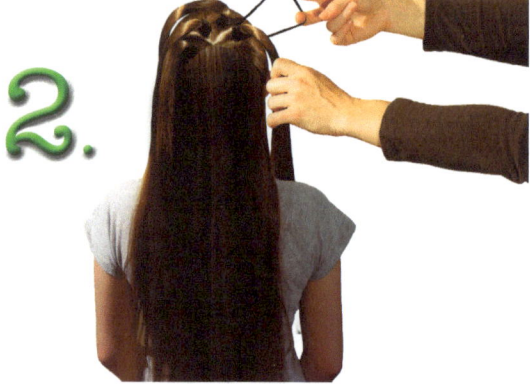

2.

Use covered rubber bands to create multiple ponytails. Leave out the cascade.

All the examples below use multiple Ponytails. Some are just the tails braided and some are pinned up into buns.

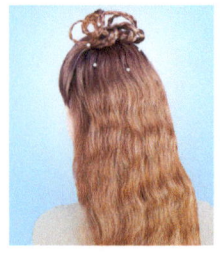
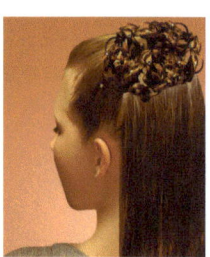
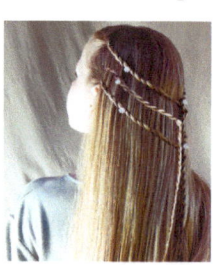
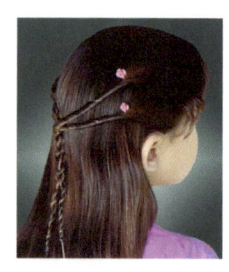
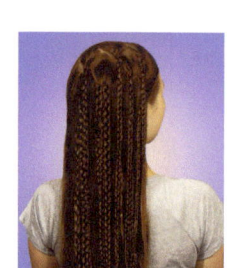

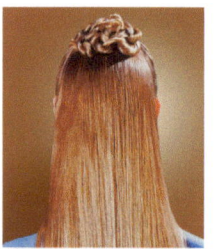
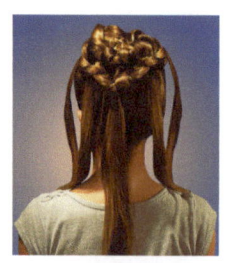
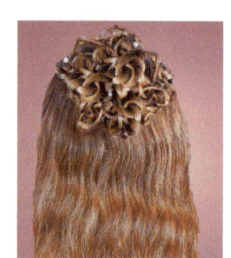
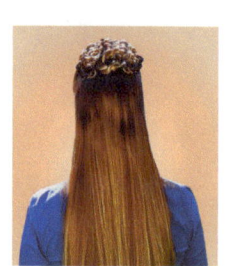

Would you open any of these with a feather loose or blossom?

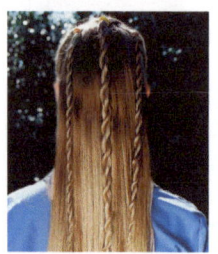
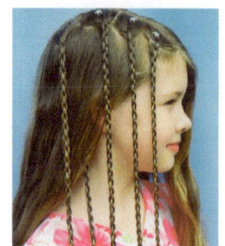
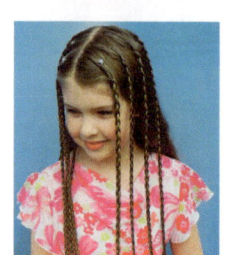
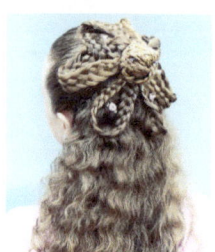

Cascade

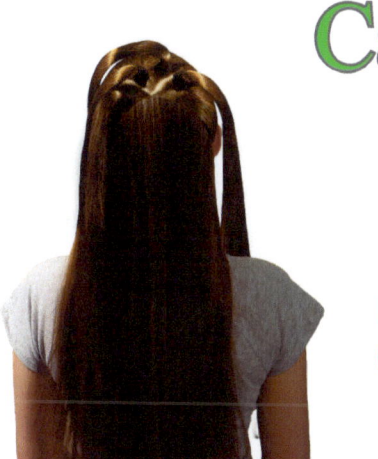

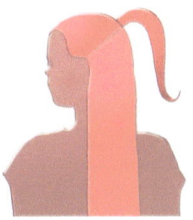

3. Once the ponytails are placed right where you want them, choose a number of strands to braid with.

After the number of strands has been chosen, decide how many braids will be made.

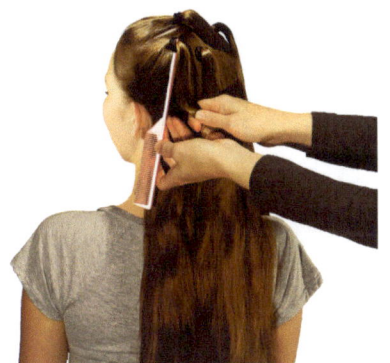

4.

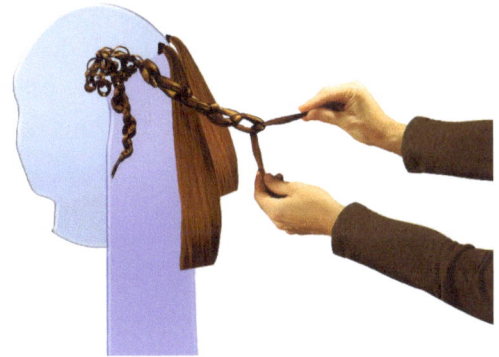

Finally, determine if those braids will hang down or be pinned up.

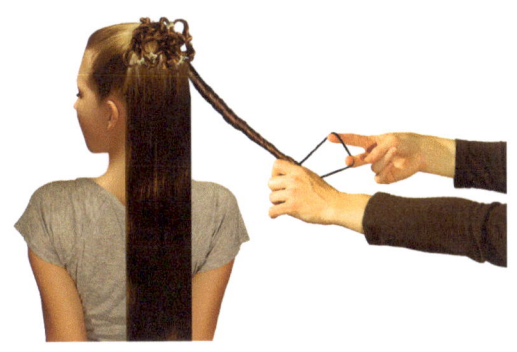

5.

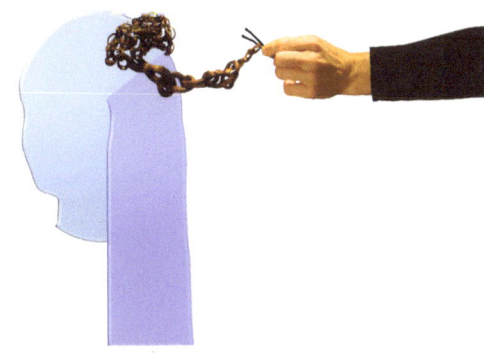

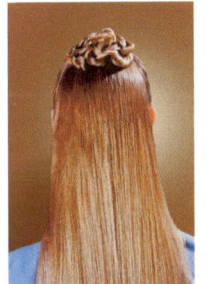

6.

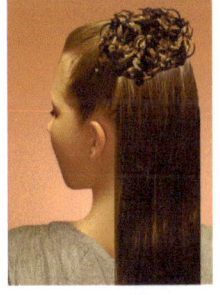

Review

What is a Cascaded Tail?

When you create cascaded tails, you may make one or 100 tails. It doesn't matter where you place the braids as long as half of the hair is left out to create a cascade.

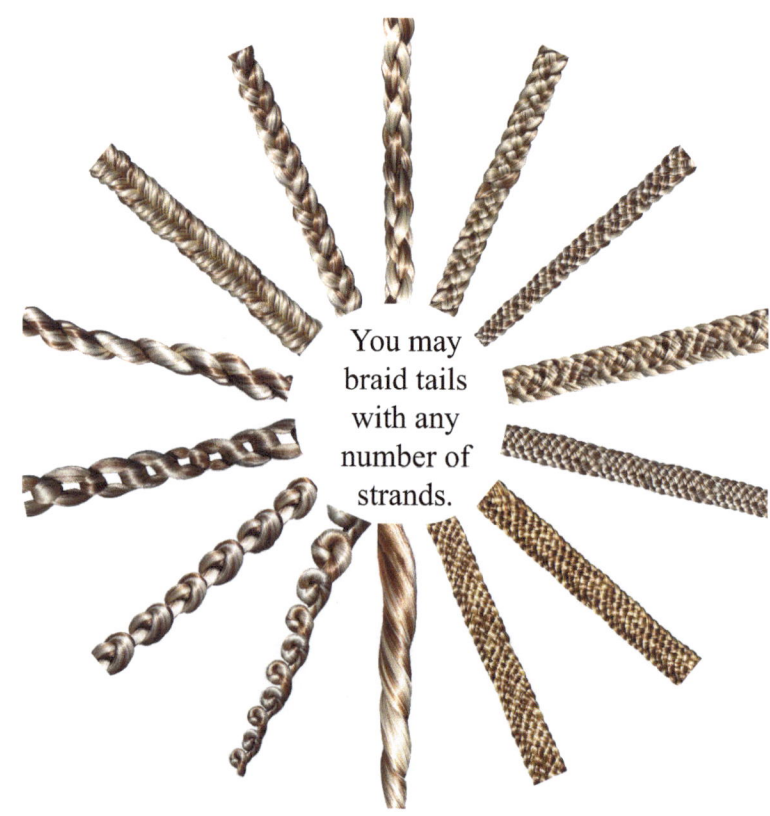

You may braid tails with any number of strands.

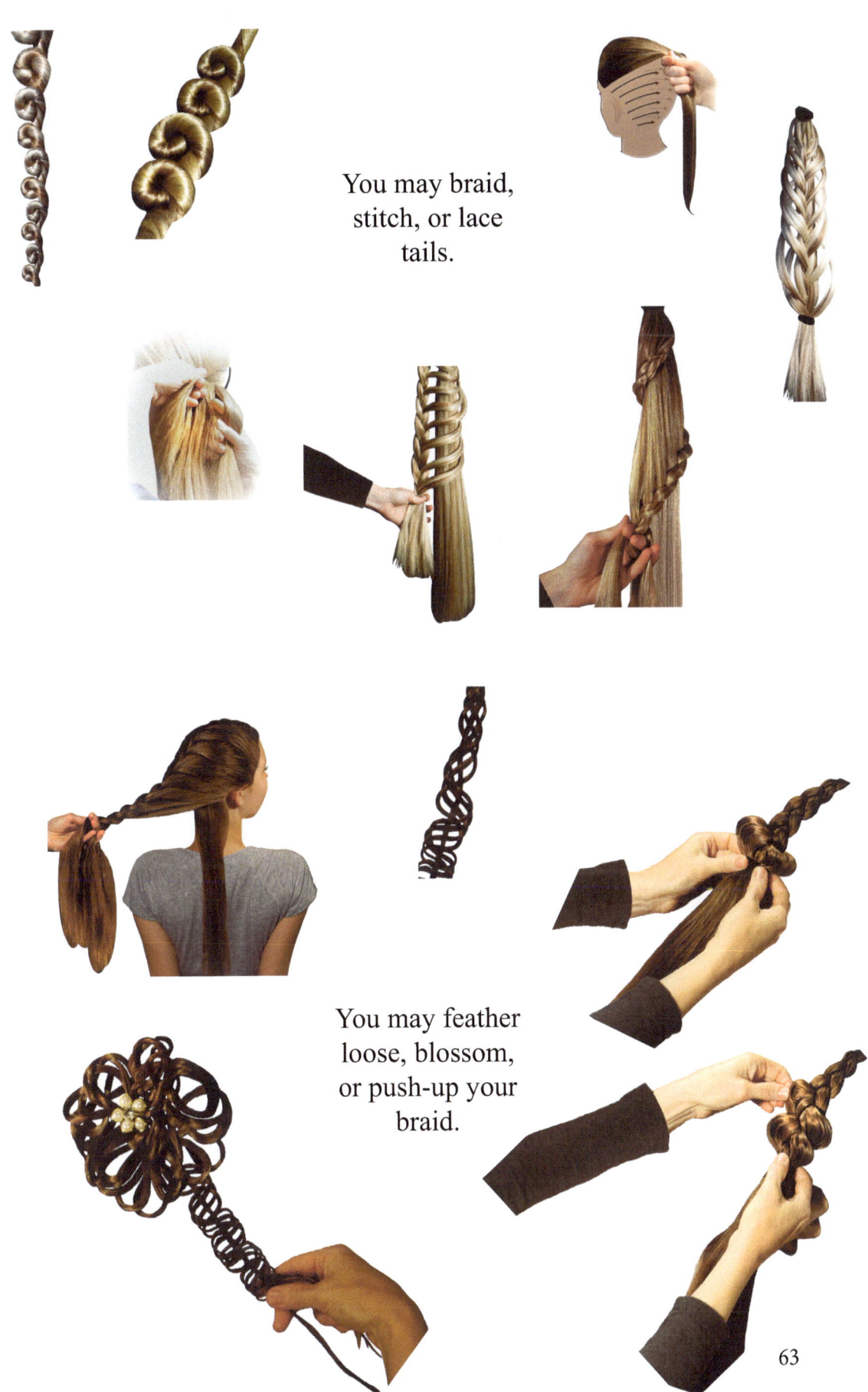

You may braid,
stitch, or lace
tails.

You may feather
loose, blossom,
or push-up your
braid.

63

Examples

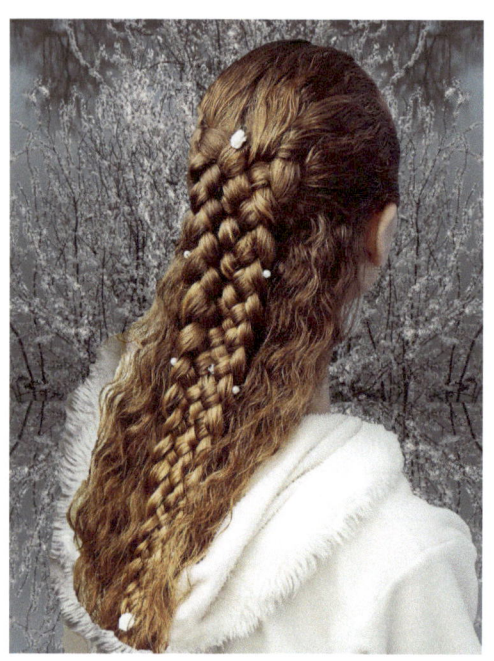
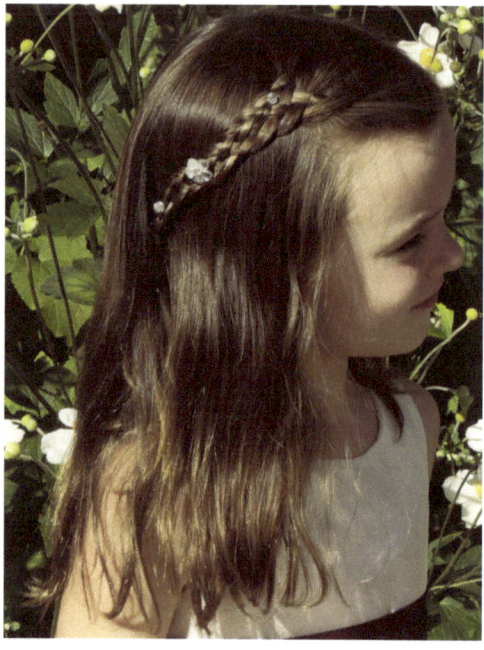
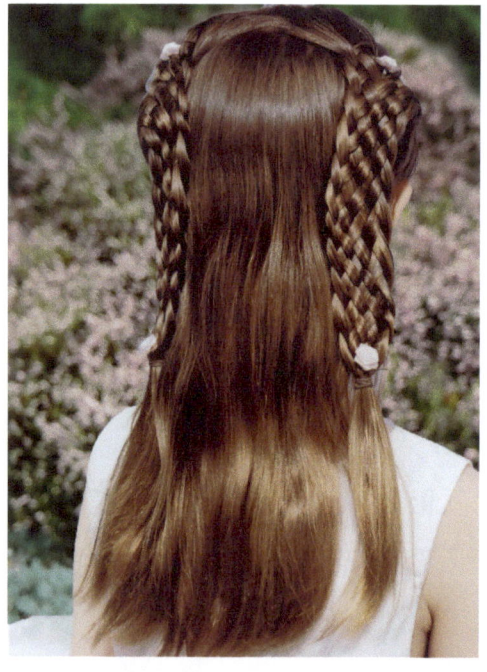
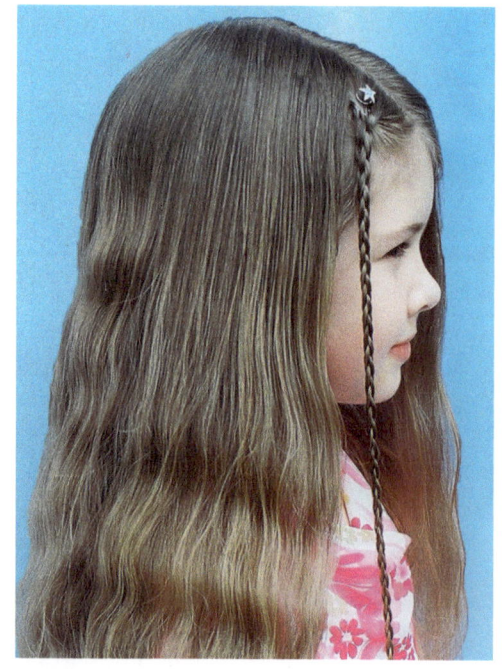

Examples

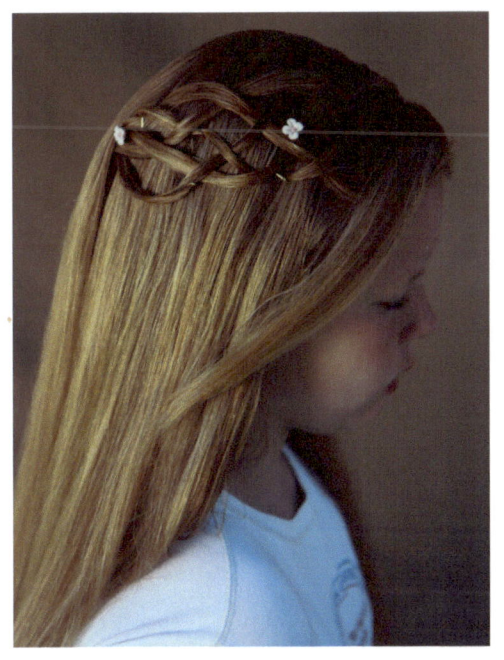
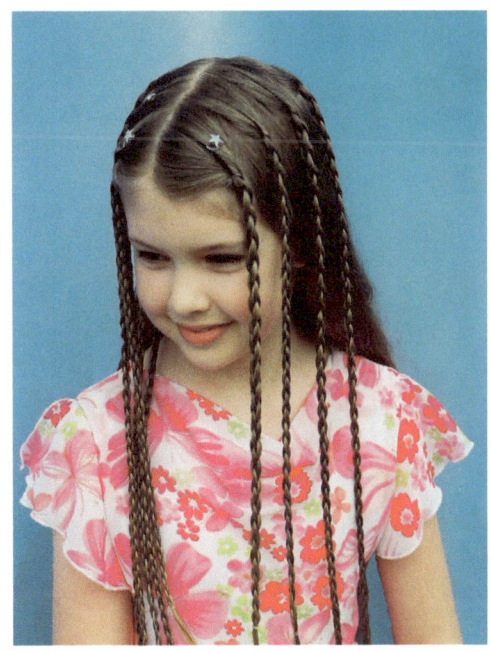
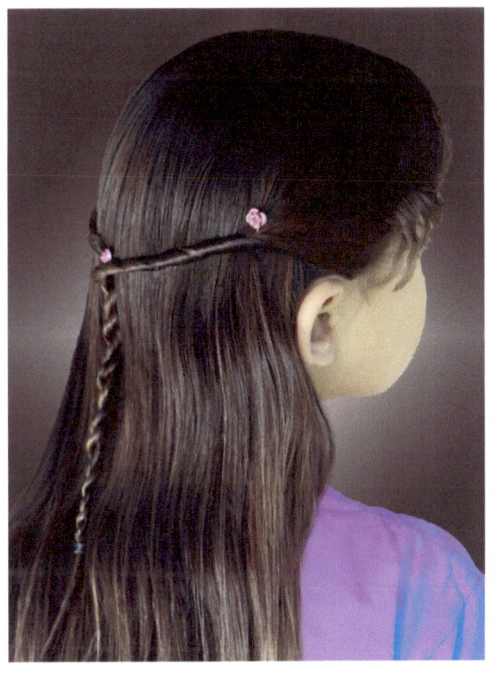
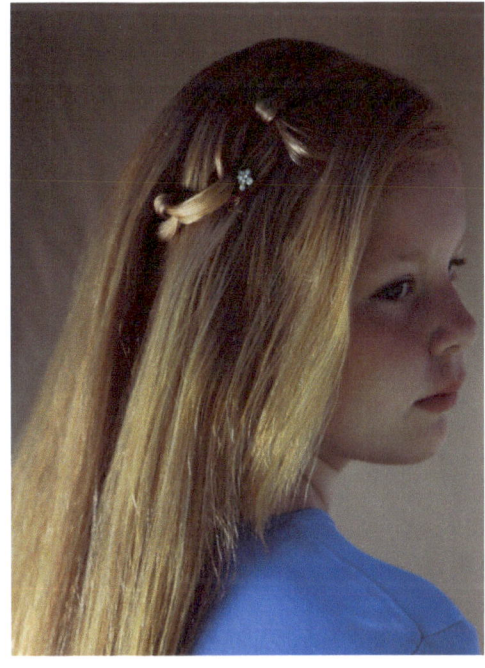

Cascade Accented Tails

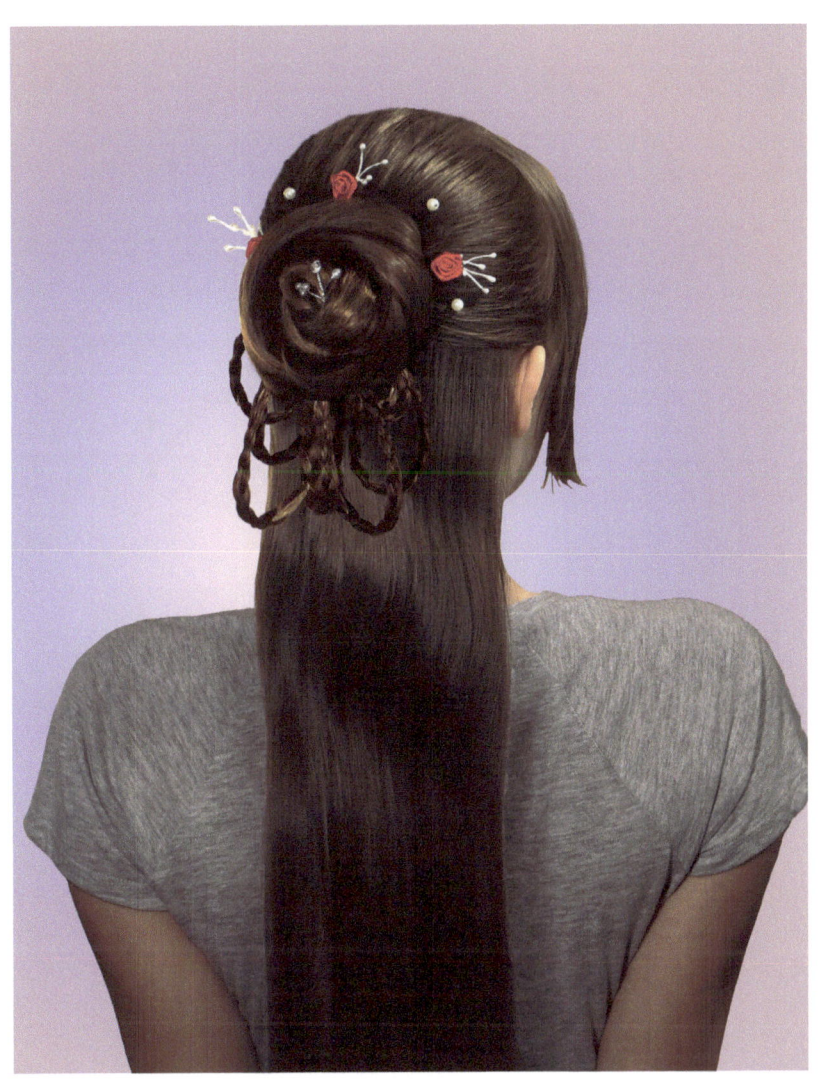

Cascade and Accent Placement

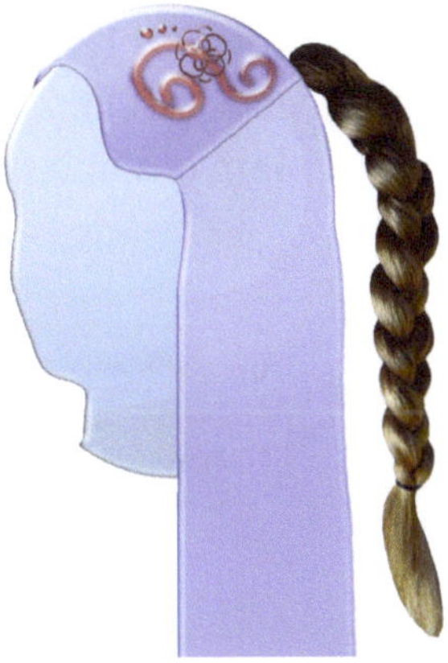

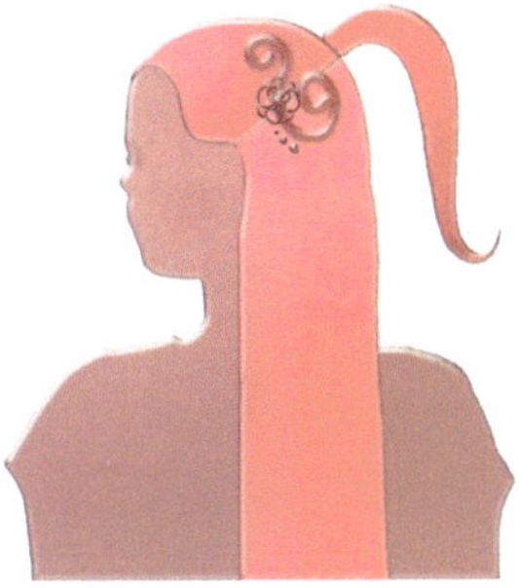

High Pony	High Side Pony	High Pigtails

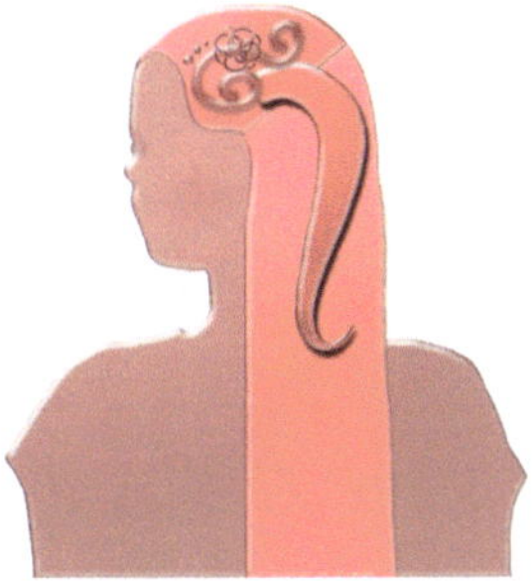

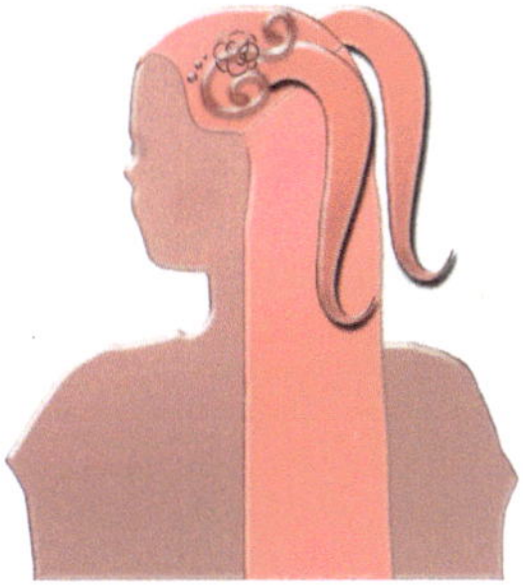

The Icons above are suggestions of a few common placements for a tail with cascade and accent. This is a small book and I will let you use your creativity to come up with the other placements. For more suggestions, review the previous sections as any style can be revised into a cascade. Also, accents may be added to any hairstyle.

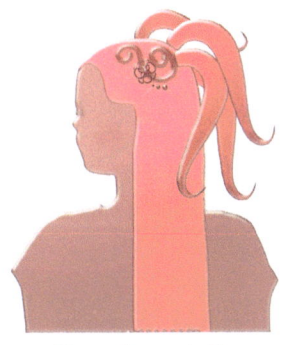

Four Ponytails

Accented Cascade

Make one tail or make 100 tails. It doesn't matter where you place the braids as long as half of the hair is left out. One or several slivers of hair are used to create accents. Accents add a decorative flare to any hairstyle including just a plain old unbraided ponytail.

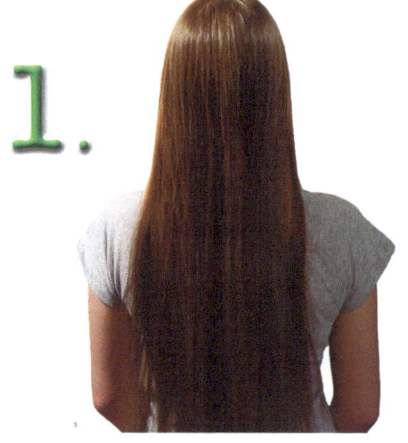

1.

Begin with clean, brushed hair.

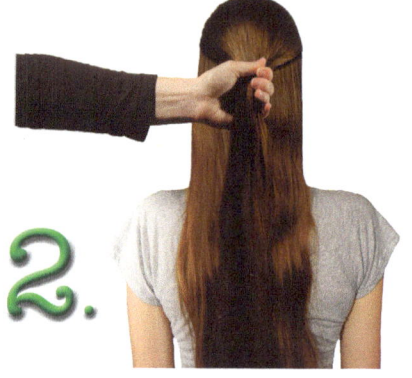

2.

Use a covered rubber band to place part of the hair into a ponytail. Leave out the cascade and accent hair.

All the examples below are tails with both cascade and an accent. The tails are braided and pinned up.

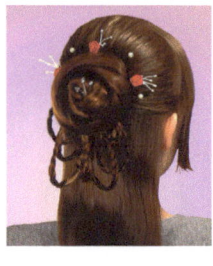
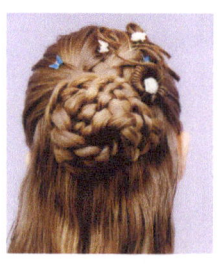
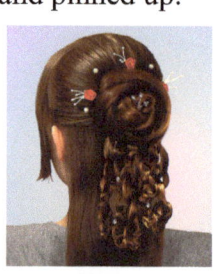
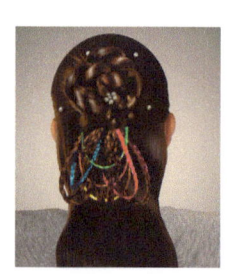

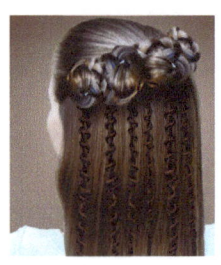
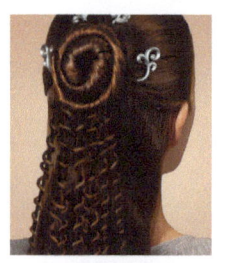
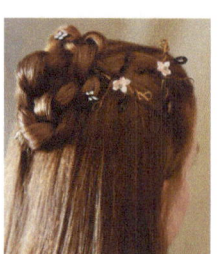
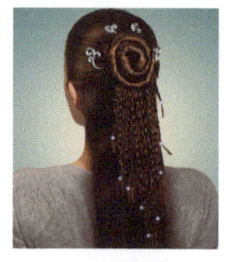
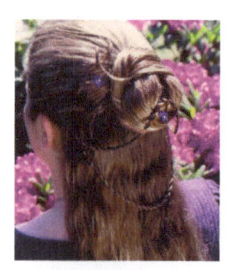

Would you open any of these with a feather loose or blossom?

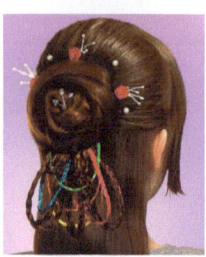
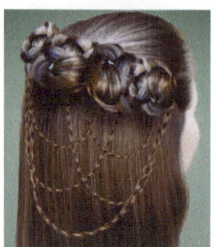
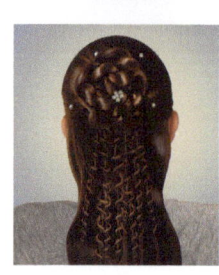
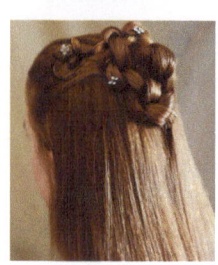

70

Accented Cascade

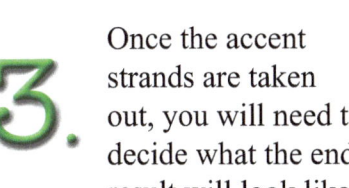

I will take accents from the cascade for these examples.

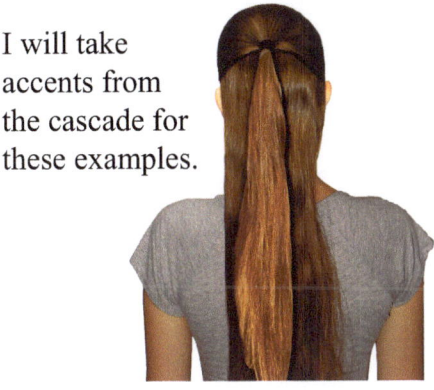

3. Once the accent strands are taken out, you will need to decide what the end result will look like.

Will you braid the ponytail? If so, with how many strands and how many braids? Will they hang down or be pinned up?

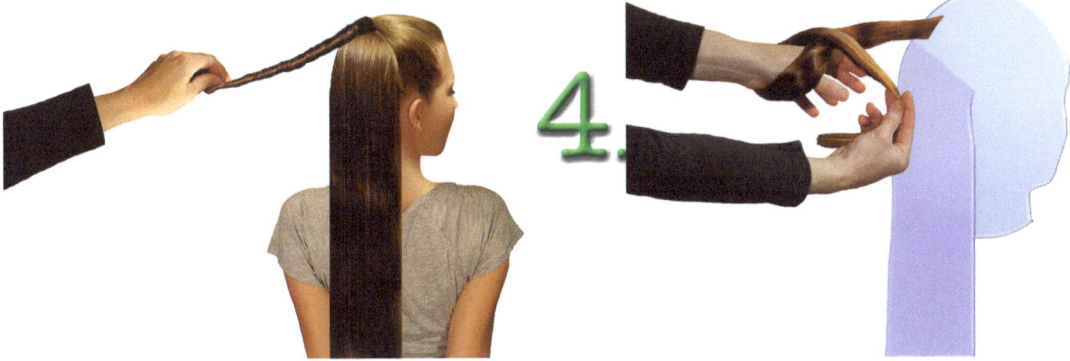

4.

What accent will be used and how many of them will you be making?

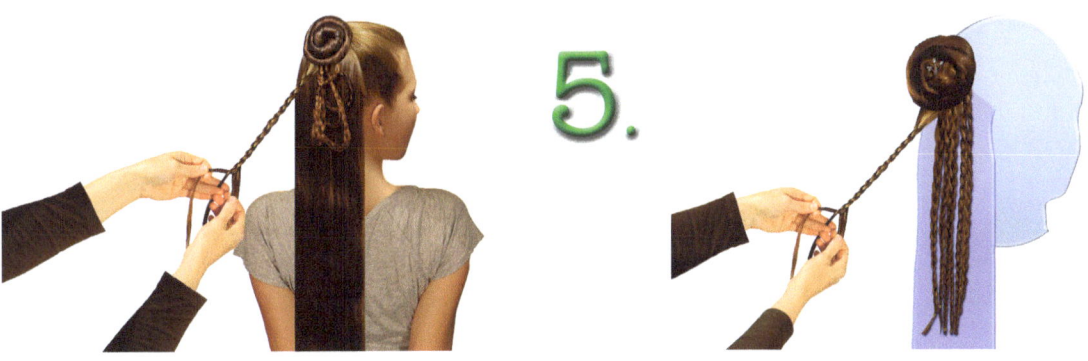

5.

Decide if the accents will hang down or be pinned up.

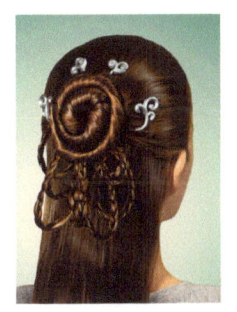

6.

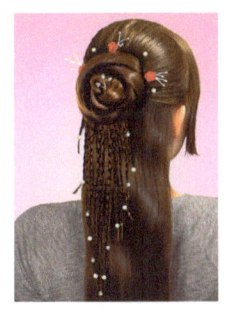

Accented Cascade

Make one tail or make 100 tails. It doesn't matter where you place the braids as long as half of the hair is left out. One or several slivers of hair are used to create accents. Accents add a decorative flare to any hairstyle including just a plain old unbraided ponytail.

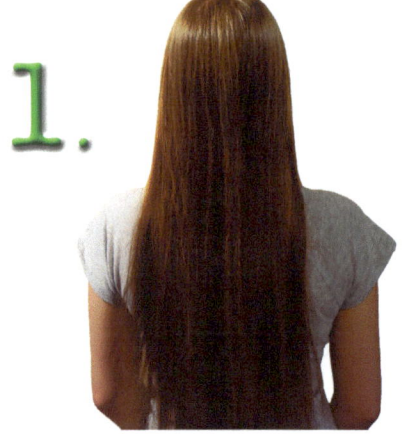

1.

Begin with clean, brushed hair.

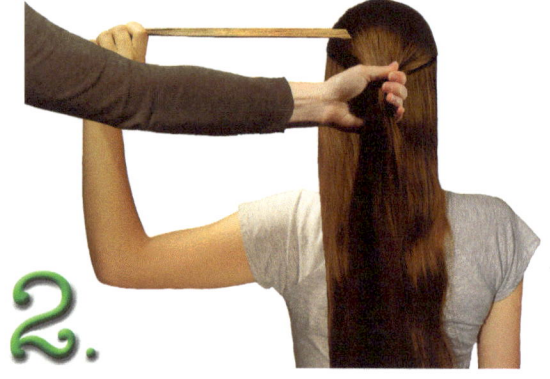

2.

Use a covered rubber band to place part of the hair into a ponytail. Leave out the cascade and accent hair.

All the examples below are tails with both cascade and an accent. The tails are braided and left down.

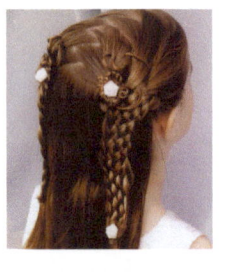
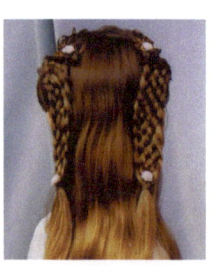
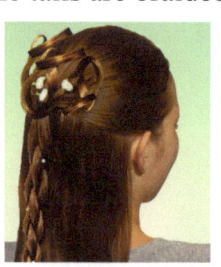
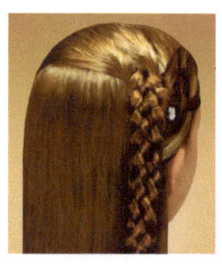
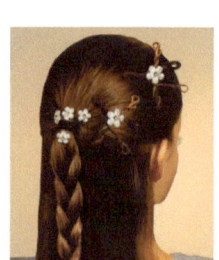

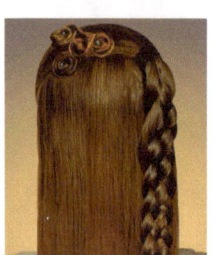
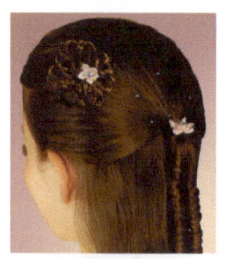
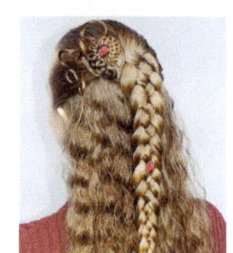
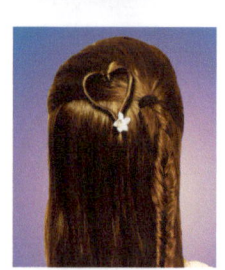

Would you open any of these with a feather loose or blossom?

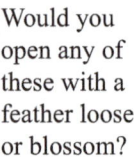
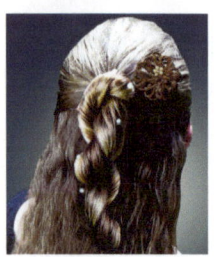
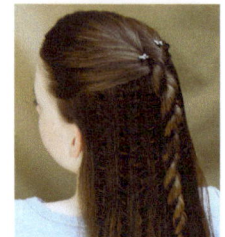
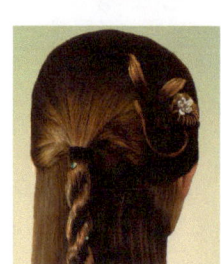
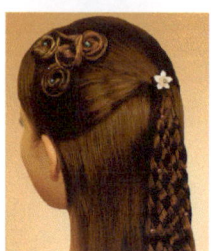

Accented Cascade

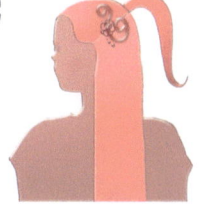

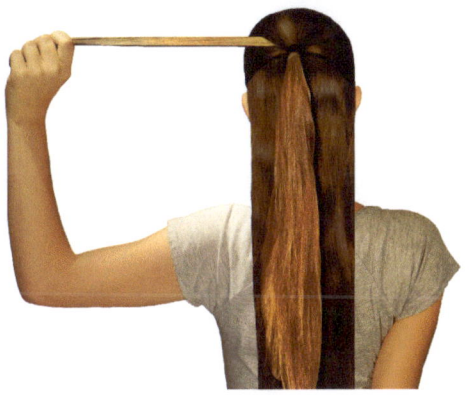

3. Once you have your accent strands taken out, you will need to decide what the end result will look like.

Will you braid the ponytail? If so, with how many strands and how many braids? Will they hang down or be pinned up?

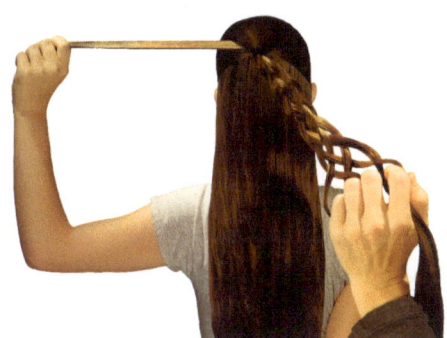

4.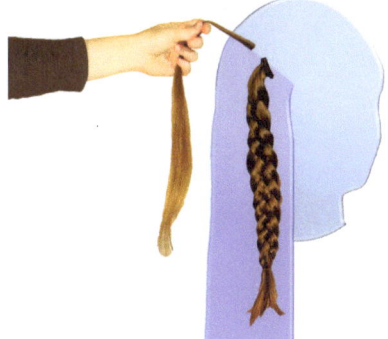

What accent will be used and how many of them will you be making?

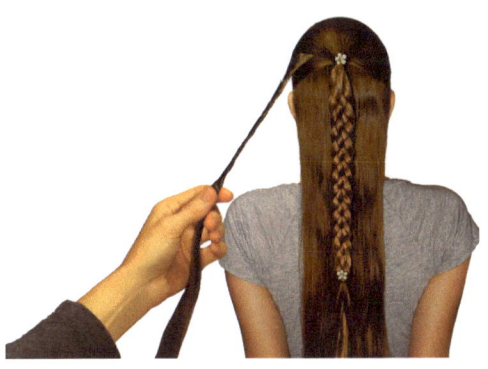

5.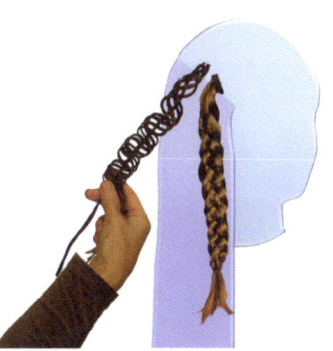

Decide if the accents will hang down or be pinned up.

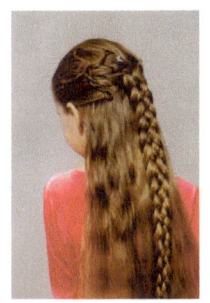

6.

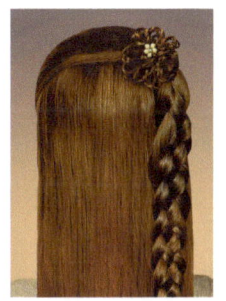

Review

What is a Cascade Accented Tail?

When you create a cascaded tail with accents, you make one tail or 100 tails. It doesn't matter where you place the braids as long as half of the hair is left out. One or several slivers of hair are used to create accents. Accents add a decorative flare to any hairstyle including just a plain old unbraided ponytail.

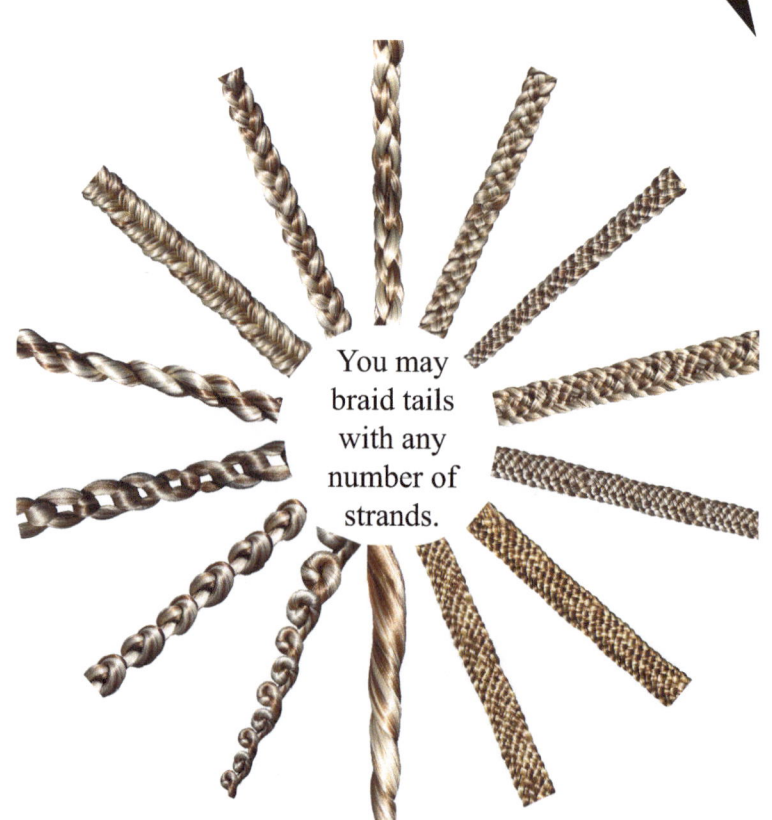

You may braid tails with any number of strands.

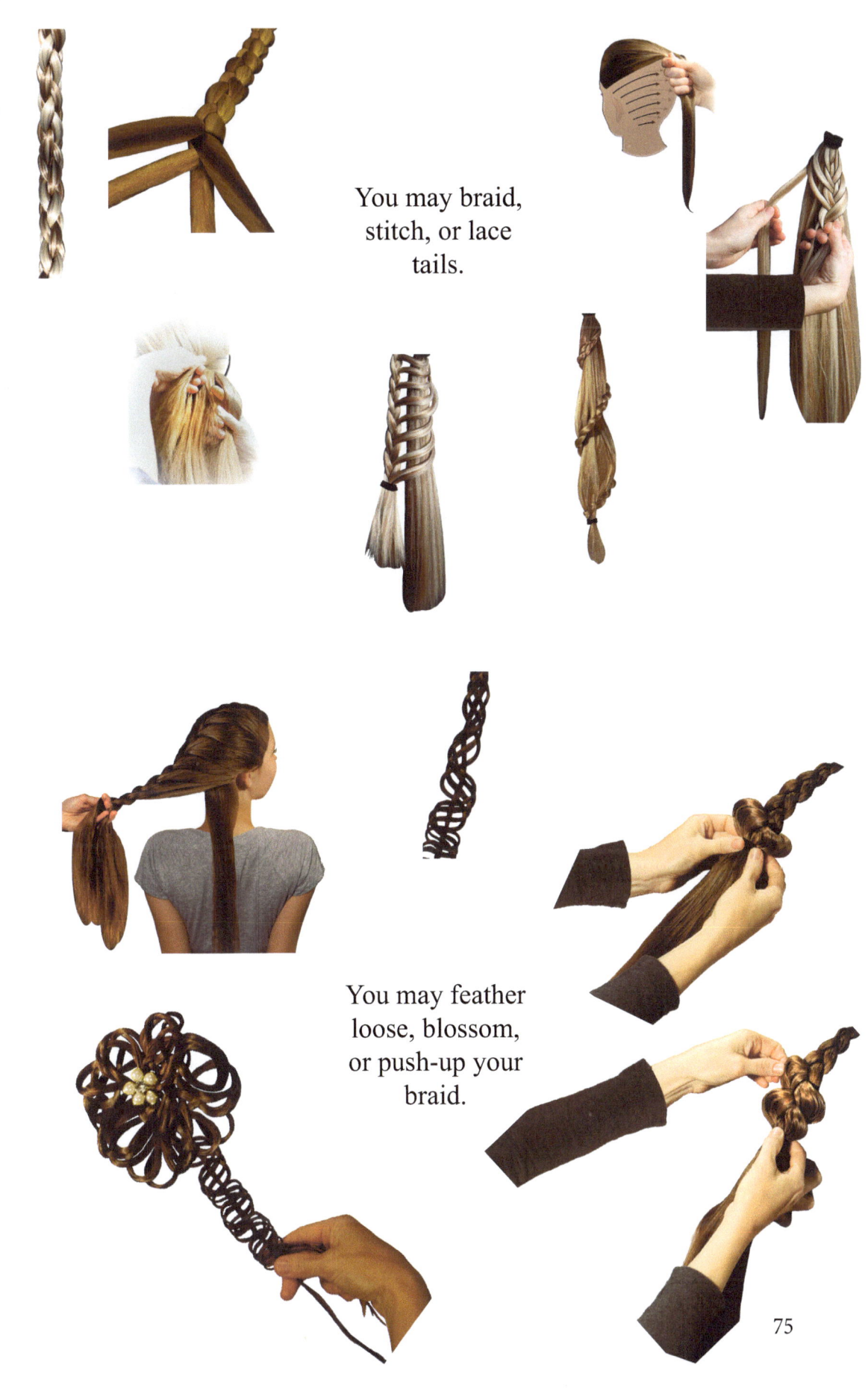

You may braid,
stitch, or lace
tails.

You may feather
loose, blossom,
or push-up your
braid.

75

Examples

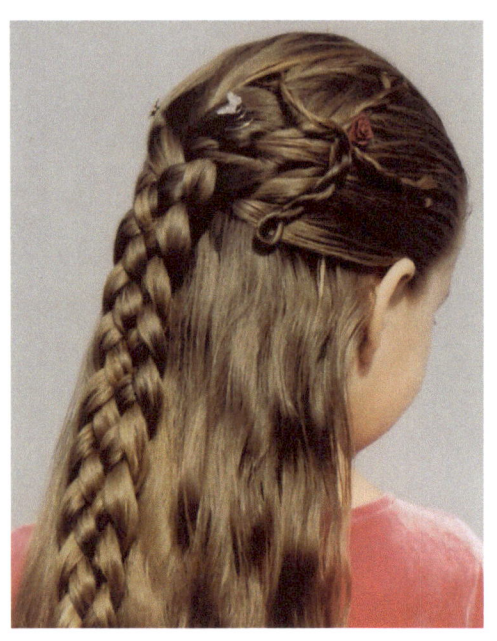
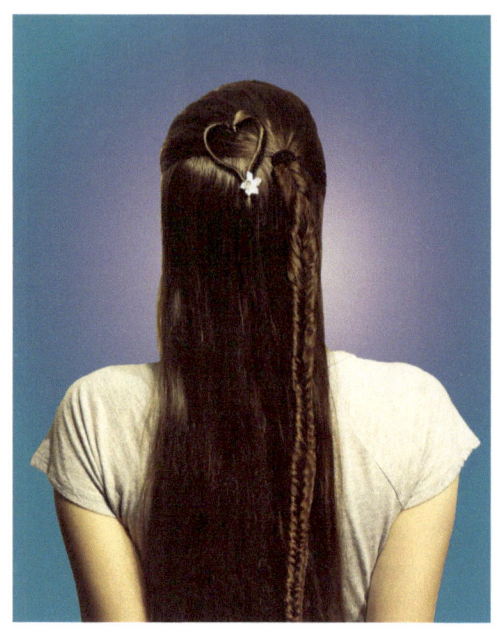

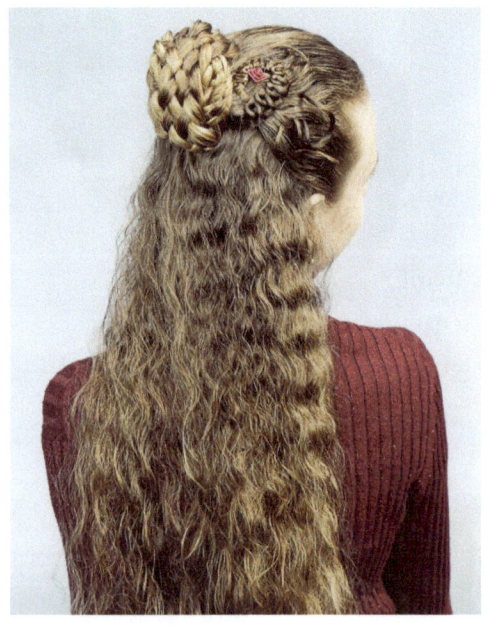
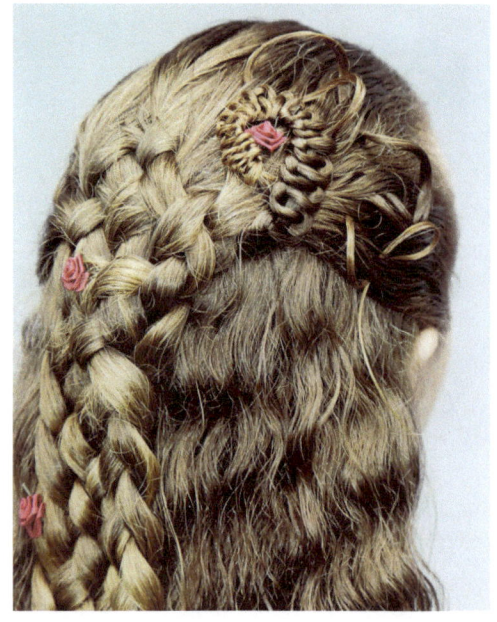

Examples

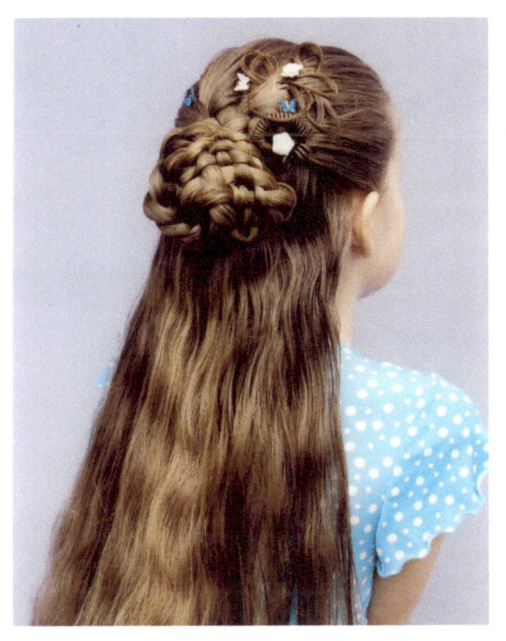
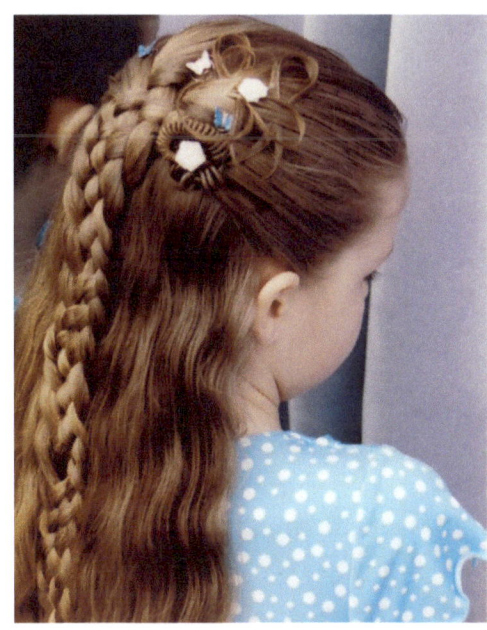
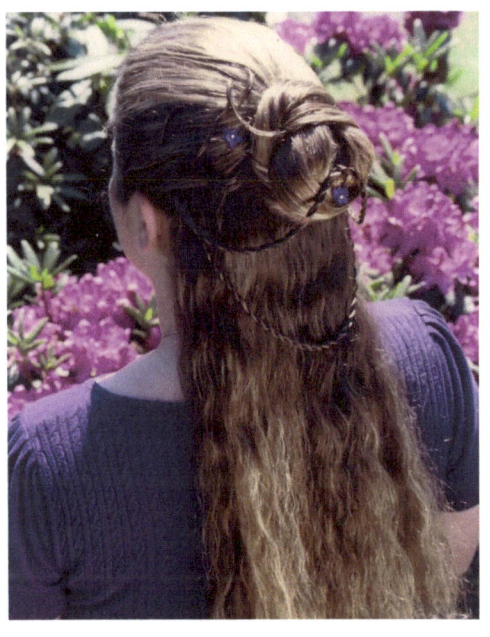
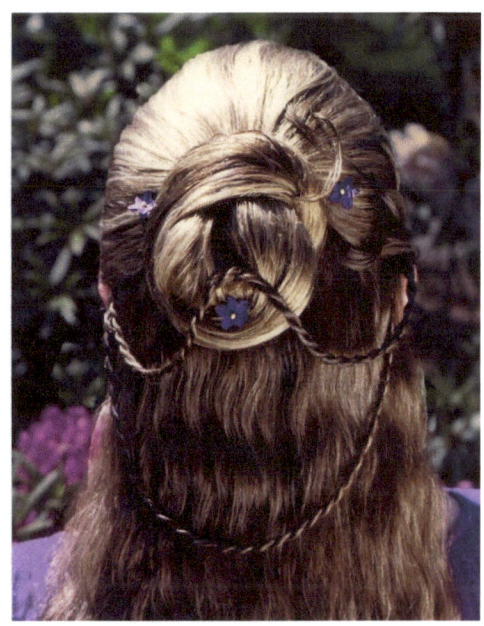

Summary

Summarizing my approach to hairstyling with braids is a complicated task. I could over simplify this section and say that only three things are needed to create hairstyles.

1. Ways: Most braids are created with a three-strand braid. Instead, apply the other twenty plus ways to braid. It is possible to find information on one-strands through nine-strands in ebooks, online and in printed books.

2. Forms: There are so many shapes available to utilize in your hairstyling extravaganza. The shapes I use are not the only ones. And don't forget, you can make up your own.

3. Accents: Accents are the prettiest part of a hairstyle. No single person can define what may be used as accents. Don't be boring like me and use the same ones over and over.

As you can see from my books, this is not a good summary. How are you supposed to use these three components to make a hairstyle? Especially knowing Ways has so many options like Stitching, Lacing, Tapering, and Braiding. All I can say is start by choosing a Form and braid that Form with all the Ways you can. See how it changes as the number of strands change. Then, add Accents as you feel comfortable. This will help you begin to dream about hairstyles.

As you apply this to all shapes, you will find yourself understanding the art. Reading will not be able to give you the confidence to create great beauty. Only practice will be able to do this. It is a painfully slow process and the first dozen tries will make you want to give up.

Then, there is that pesky business of what is possible during the braiding process: Feather Loose, Blossom, Push-up, Ladder, Waterfall, Cascade, and Basic. When and how do you apply these techniques? You may mimic other peoples hairstyles and what they do. That is great. But, I urge you to keep the whole plan in mind while you are learning and applying these techniques.

Apply them everywhere possible (all the Ways and Forms). Be brave enough to make up some pretty silly and unattractive hairstyles. This is when and where you will learn how to use these techniques, not by copying other peoples hairstyles.

What is this Braider Creator I keep talking about? It is a wheel that is available on my website (www.findingbraids.com). Download it. Assemble it. This wheel points out hairstyle possibilities. The arrow resides above the four components of a style: Ways, Forms, Accents, and Basic or Cascade.

Whoa, what is up with Basic and Cascade? I thought there were only three things. Sorry, Basic and Cascades are part of Forms but separated out on the wheel.

Give the wheel to a dozen people and have them all line up the same items. When they create the suggested style, you will be surprised how the "same" style varies. We all interpret what we see and hear differently because of our unique backgrounds and what we know individually.

My goal is to teach people how to create hairstyles so that the world is filled with beauty. Start out copying styles in order to learn, but as you get comfortable, use the wheel to start making up your own hairstyles. If you only copy hairstyles, then we all look the same. Unleash your creativity. Eventually, people will start copying your hairstyles.

Someday, the wheel will be too limiting for your imagination. That will be a glorious moment. I look forward to it.

Raychel

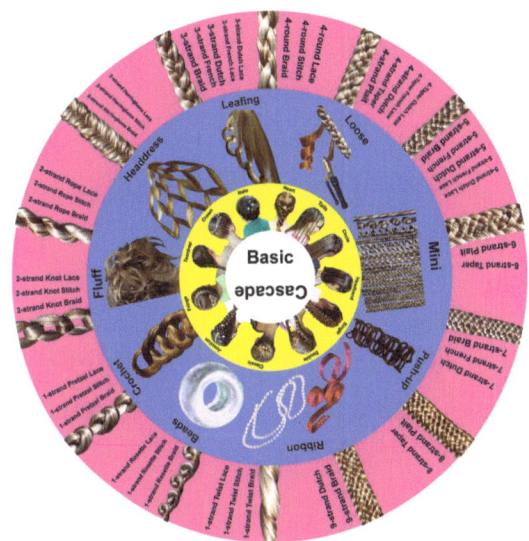

How to use this book

This book is assuming you already know how to braid or have the book <u>A Different Approach to Hairbraiding: French Braiding and More</u>.

This book expands upon the **Tail** section of Chapter Two in <u>A Different Approach to Hairbraiding: French Braiding and More</u>.

Chapter Two in <u>A Different Approach to Hairbraiding: French Braiding and More</u> teaches 12 Forms: **Tails**, Headband, Circle, Single, Double, Junction, Classic, Teardrop, Fringe, Crown, Halo, Heart.

There are 11 other books to this mini series: Headband, Circle, Single, Double, Junction, Classic, Teardrop, Fringe, Crown, Halo, Heart.

So why didn't I just include all this information in the first book <u>A Different Approach to Hairbraiding: French Braiding and More</u>? Because the book would have been nearly 1,500 pages long. And it is already huge at 500 pages.

So how does someone use this book anyway? If you don't have the first book, you can learn how to braid from a parent, friend, video, internet, youtube, or spend hours playing with hair until something comes out looking like a braid. Then memorize that braid and apply it to the shape in this book <u>Tails</u>. This book shows you how to create many hairstyles from a tail form. Even with your one made-up braid, you can create hundreds of hairstyles using this book.

If you do know how to braid, apply all of your braiding knowledge to the tails form. You will be able to create thousands of styles by mixing and matching the number of strands you braid with, and the four options shown on page nine, and all the accents.

Good luck and have fun creating!

Braiding a Tail

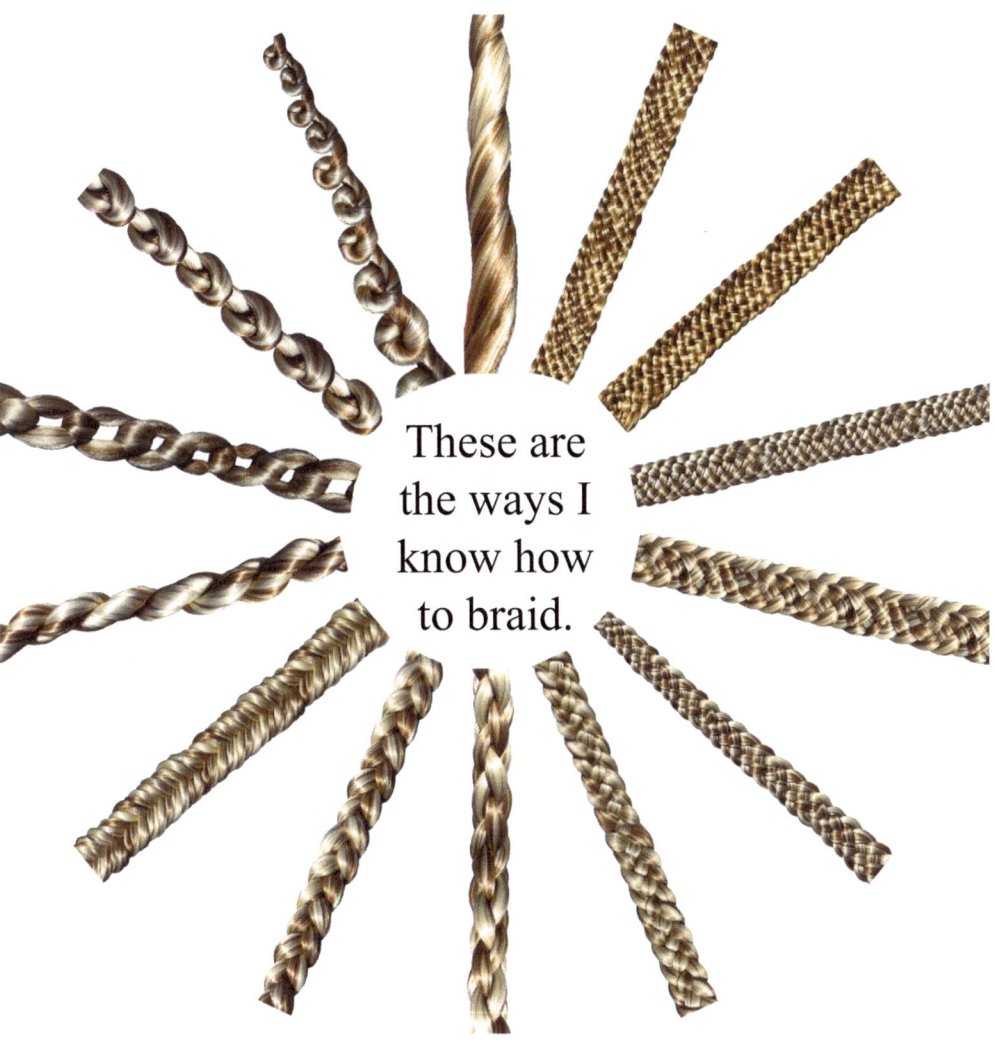

These are the ways I know how to braid.

There are so many ways to braid. This book does not teach how to braid these ways. This book shows how incredibly versatile the tail form is. It is not possible to show all the numbers of strands with the four different options shown on page nine with all the accents. So we will just go over a few and I hope that you will be able to fill in the gaps on your own.

Links

www.findingbraids.com
frenchbraidsbytwistedsisters.com
www.martinparsons.com
www.aquage.com
www.patrick-cameron.com
www.youtube.com/raychelnorberg
www.youtube.com/ViriYueMoon
www.youtube.com/lilithedarkmoon
www.youtube.com/womenbeauty1
www.youtube.com/cinthiatruong

There are so many great braiding books out there, these are my favorites:

Braids and More, by Andrea Jeffery, 1991
Braids and Updos, by Jamie Rines Jones, 1996
Trenzas Plaits 2, by Susana Burgos, 2002
Great Braids, by Thomas Hardy, 1997

Biography

Melanie Mundy was my first mentor. She is the most meticulous braider I have ever met. I was blessed to have her as a teacher.

During the years I lived in Oregon I attended cosmetology school to get my barber's license. I came across a hairdresser named Martin Parsons. For months, I sat in front of my television absorbing all of his videos. The man is brilliant.

The magic of the Aquage Team caught my attention. I trained with them, carefully learning all I could. Luis Alvarez is a genius.

After digesting and blending this knowledge I now do unique hairstyles for my clients.

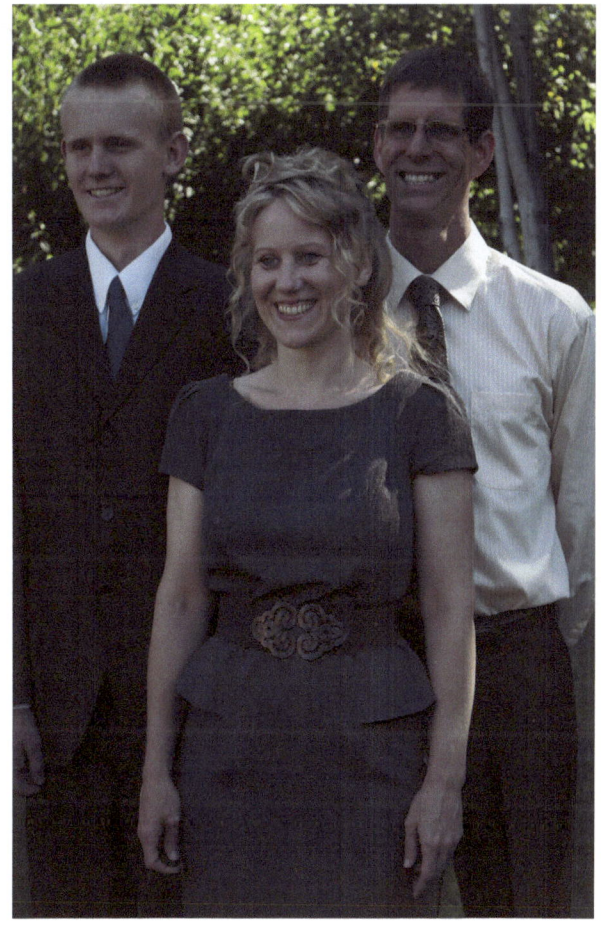

I enjoy volunteering my skill to local community events. My favorites in the past have been high school plays, community theaters, girl scout troops, fashion shows, and giving back to the beauty schools. I taught classes at the community college in Corvallis. Gift certificates make it easy for me to donate to local fund raisers.

My work is a happy work. I love what I do. It never crossed my mind that I would be a hairstylist when I grew up. When I was a kid I wanted to be a ballerina and when I was a teenager I wanted to be a geologist. Now, I am a happy hair artist.

www.ingramcontent.com/pod-product-compliance
Lightning Source LLC
Chambersburg PA
CBHW041458280526
45792CB00004B/1050